W0017923

ANNALS *of* THE NEW YORK ACADEMY OF SCIENCES

DIRECTOR AND EXECUTIVE EDITOR
Douglas Braaten

PROJECT MANAGER
Steven E. Bohall

The New York Academy of Sciences
7 World Trade Center
250 Greenwich Street, 40th Floor
New York, NY 10007-2157

annals@nyas.org
www.nyas.org/annals

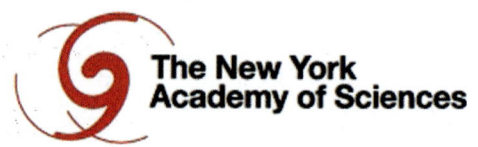

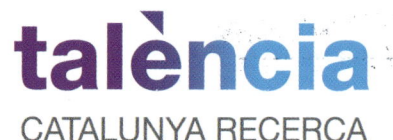

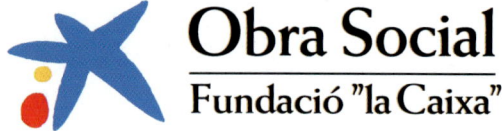

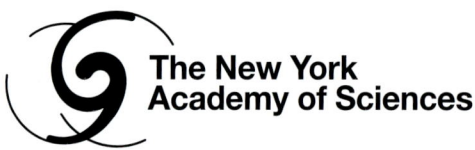

Published by Blackwell Publishing
On behalf of The New York Academy of Sciences

Boston, Massachusetts
2010

ANNALS *of* THE NEW YORK ACADEMY OF SCIENCES

VOLUME
1210

ISSUE

Toward Personalized Medicine for Cancer

This volume presents manuscripts stemming from the conference entitled "Towards Personalized Cancer Medicine," held on May 19–21, 2010 in Barcelona, Spain. The conference was presented by the New York Academy of Sciences, Talència, and Foundation Obra Social La Caixa; and supported by the Mushett Family Foundation, Roche (Gold sponsors); Amgen S.A., Life Technologies, MedImmune, Ramon Areces Foundation (Silver sponsors); Cepheid, Ferrer InCode, IkerChem S.L., LIFE Biosystems AG, Millennium Pharmaceuticals–The Takeda Oncology Company, Novartis (Bronze sponsors); Affymetrix, Agilent Technologies, Bayer Schering Pharma, Biocat (the BioRegion of Catalonia), Catalan Institute of Oncology, Cell Signaling Technology, Inc., Laboratorio de Análisis Dr. Echevarne, Pangaea Biotech S.A., USP Instituto Universitario Dexeus (Academy Friends); and by grants from ImClone Systems, a wholly owned subsidiary of Eli Lilly and Company; and from the National Cancer Institute and the National Human Genome Research Institute.

TABLE OF CONTENTS

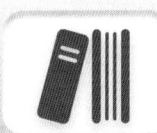

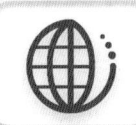

Ann. N.Y. Acad. Sci. ISSN 0077-8923

ANNALS OF THE NEW YORK ACADEMY OF SCIENCES
Issue: *Toward Personalized Medicine for Cancer*

New cancer targets emerging from studies of the Von Hippel-Lindau tumor suppressor protein

William G. Kaelin, Jr.

Howard Hughes Medical Institute, Dana-Farber Cancer Institute and Brigham and Women's Hospital, Harvard Medical School, Boston, Massachusetts

Address for correspondence: William G. Kaelin, Jr., Professor of Medicine, Dana-Farber Cancer Institute, 44 Binney Street, Mayer 457, Boston, MA 02115. william_kaelin@dfci.harvard.edu

Inactivation of the von Hippel-Lindau tumor suppressor protein (pVHL) causes the most common form of kidney cancer. pVHL is part of a complex that polyubiquitinates the alpha subunit of the heterodimeric transcription factor HIF. In the presence of oxygen, HIF1α is prolyl hydroxylated by EglN1 (also called PHD2); this modification recruits pVHL, which then targets HIF1α for proteasomal degradation. In hypoxic or pVHL-defective cells, HIF1α accumulates, binds to HIF1β, and transcriptionally activates genes such as VEGF. VEGF inhibitors and mTOR inhibitors, which indirectly affect HIF, are now approved for the treatment of kidney cancer. EglN1 is a 2-oxoglutarate–dependent dioxygenase; such enzymes can be inhibited with drug-like small molecules and EglN1 inhibitors are currently being tested for the treatment of anemia. EglN2 (PHD1) and EglN3 (PHD3), which are EglN1 paralogs, appear to play HIF-independent roles in cell proliferation and apoptosis, respectively, and are garnering interest as potential cancer targets. A number of JmjC-containing proteins, including RBP2 and PLU-1, are 2-oxoglutarate–dependent dioxygenases that demethylate histones. Preclinical data suggest that inhibition of RBP2 or PLU-1 would suppress tumor growth.

Keywords: cancer; tumor suppressor protein; transcription factor

Individuals bearing a germline, loss of function, mutation of the von Hippel-Lindau (*VHL*) tumor suppressor gene, which resides on chromosome 3p25, develop von Hippel-Lindau disease.[1] This hereditary cancer syndrome is characterized by an increased risk of developing a number of tumors, including hemangioblastomas of the retina, cerebellum, and spinal cord, clear cell renal carcinomas, pheochromocytomas, endolymphatic sac tumors, pancreatic islet cell tumors, and cyst adenomas of the broad ligament or epididymis. Tumor development in this setting is linked to inactivation or loss of the remaining wild-type *VHL* allele in a susceptible cell. Biallelic *VHL* inactivation, either due to somatic mutations or hypermethylation, is also common in sporadic clear cell renal carcinomas, which are the most common form of kidney cancer.

The *VHL* gene product, pVHL, is the substrate recognition component of an E3 ubiquitin ligase complex that, in the presence of oxygen, directly interacts with the alpha subunit of the heterodimeric hypoxia-inducible factor (HIF) transcription factor and orchestrates its polyubiquitination and destruction.[2] When oxygen levels are low, or pVHL is defective, HIFα accumulates, dimerizes with its partner protein HIFβ (also called the aryl hydrocarbon receptor nuclear translocator or ARNT), and transcriptionally activates 100–200 genes, many of which promote survival in a hypoxic environment including genes that promote angiogenesis, erythropoiesis, and maintenance of energy homeostasis through changes in metabolism.

Recognition of HIFα by pVHL requires that the former be hydroxylated on one (or both) of two prolyl residues by members of the EglN (also called PHD) family of prolyl hydroxylases[2] (Fig. 1). This reaction is intrinsically oxygen-dependent because the oxygen atom of the hydroxyl group is derived from molecular oxygen and because the oxygen Kms for these enzymes are just slightly above that encountered in normal tissues.[3,4] As a result, decrements in oxygen availability lead to decreased HIFα

doi: 10.1111/j.1749-6632.2010.05781.x
Ann. N.Y. Acad. Sci. 1210 (2010) 1–7 © 2010 The New York Academy of Sciences.

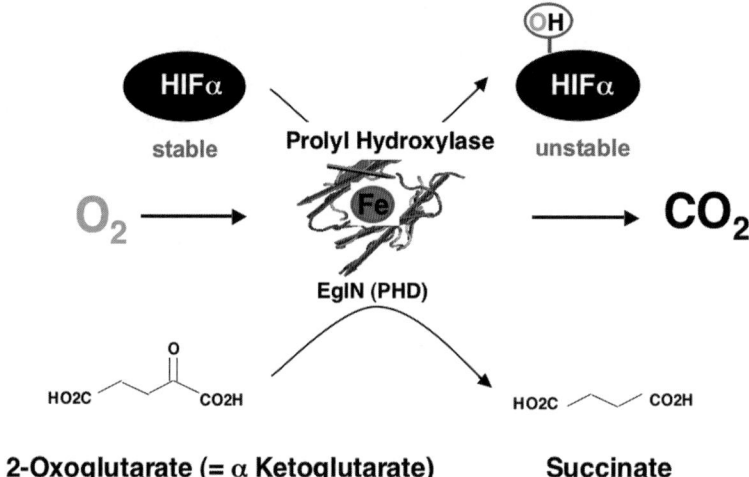

Figure 1. Prolyl hydroxylation of HIFα. When oxygen is present, HIFα becomes hydroxylated on one (or both) of two prolyl residues by members of the EglN (also called PHD) family in a reaction that requires ferrous iron and 2-oxoglutarate. Hydroxylation of HIFα, which targets it for degradation, is coupled to the decarboxylation of 2-oxoglutarate to succinate.

hydroxylation. In addition to oxygen, these enzymes require ferrous iron, ascorbate, and 2-oxoglutarate (also called α-ketoglutarate). The latter is decarboxylated to succinate during the course of the hydroxylation reaction (Fig. 1).

EglN1 (also called PHD2) appears to be the primary HIF prolyl hydroxylase under normal conditions, with EglN2 and EglN3 playing compensatory roles under certain conditions.[5–7] Inactivation of EglN1 in mice leads to polycythemia, resulting from overproduction of erythropoietin by the kidney, and germline EglN1 mutations have been linked to familial polycythemia in man.[8–11] During fetal life the liver is the main source of erythropoietin production, with the kidney assuming this role shortly after birth. As a result, chronic renal failure, which affects over 20 million Americans, is often associated with chronic anemia.[12] We recently showed, however, that inactivation of all three EglN paralogs is sufficient to reactivate hepatic erythropoietin production.[13] In keeping with this, EglN inhibitory drugs can induce erythropoietin in anephric mice[14] and are currently being tested for the treatment of anemia in man.

pVHL has also been linked to other cellular activities that appear to be, at least partly, HIF-independent. For example, pVHL plays roles in maintenance of the primary cilium, microtubule stability, senescence, and apoptosis.[15,16] Many of these activities could, conceivably, contribute to the tumor suppressor activity of pVHL. Nonetheless, genotype-phenotype correlations in VHL patients suggest that deregulation of HIF contributes to the pathogenesis of clear cell renal carcinomas and hemangioblastomas (the same does not appear to be true for pheochromocytomas).[15,16] Moreover preclinical data as well as clinical observations, outlined below, strongly suggest that increased HIF activity plays a causal role in clear cell renal carcinoma.

There are three HIFα family members called HIF1α, HIF2α, and HIF3α. HIF1α is the canonical, well-studied, HIFα family member and is ubiquitiously expressed. The expression of HIF2α is more restricted and it is increasingly clear that the functions of HIF1α and HIF2α only partially overlap. For example, HIF1α and HIF2α share many, but not all, of their transcriptional targets. In addition, the two proteins differ with respect to crosstalk with other transcription factors such a c-Myc, where HIF1α potentiates, and HIF2α antagonizes, c-Myc activity in certain settings.[17,18]

pVHL-defective clear cell renal carcinomas produce HIF2α alone or both HIF1α and HIF2α.[19] Overproduction of a stabilized version of HIF2α, but not HIF1α, can override pVHL's ability to suppress tumor growth in nude mouse xenograft assays.[20,21] Conversely, eliminating HIF2α is sufficient to inhibit pVHL-defective tumor growth *in vivo*.[22,23]

In genetically engineered mouse models the phenotypes observed after pVHL inactivation appear to be largely driven by HIF2α.[24–27] Finally, the appearance of HIF2α in preneoplastic renal lesions in VHL patients heralds malignant transformation as determined by increased signs of dysplasia.[28] Collectively, these findings support an important role for HIF2α in clear cell renal carcinoma.

These considerations have prompted the preclinical and clinical testing of drugs that, directly or indirectly, inhibit HIF2α or its downstream targets for the treatment of kidney cancer. For example, human kidney cancers produce very high levels of VEGF, presumably because VEGF is a HIF target, and respond to VEGF blockade in the clinic. Indeed, four drugs that inhibit VEGF (bevacizumab) or its receptor, KDR (sunitinib, sorafenib, and pazopanib) have been approved for this indication on the basis of positive Phase 3 trial data in metastatic kidney cancer.[29–32] The rapamycin-like drugs (rapalogs) temsirolimus and everolimus, which inhibit the mTOR kinase, have also been approved for the treatment of kidney cancer.[33,34] These agents indirectly downregulate HIFα within cancer cells and probably also blunt signaling downstream of VEGF in endothelial cells. Unfortunately, rapalogs preferentially inhibit mTOR when it is part of the TORC1 complex rather than part of the TORC2 complex.[35] A recent report suggested that HIF1α is regulated by TORC1 whereas HIF2α is under the control of TORC2.[36] It will be of interest to see if second generation mTOR inhibitors that inhibit both TORC1 and TORC2 will have greater activity in kidney cancer by virtue of more effective TORC2 blockade.

Kidney cancer patients treated with VEGF inhibitors or mTOR inhibitors invariably relapse and the resistance mechanisms are poorly understood. Curative therapy for kidney cancer will almost certainly require combinations of agents that have distinct mechanisms of action and that are non-cross-resistant. New targets for kidney cancer will likely be produced by several lines of investigation. For example, state of the art genomic technologies, including high density SNP arrays, expression profiling, and exon resequencing, are being used in an attempt to identify the mutations that cooperate with pVHL loss to cause kidney cancer.[37–41] In addition, targets that, when inhibited, preferentially kill pVHL-defective cells owing to synthetic lethal interactions are being sought by exposing isogenic cell line pairs to collections of shRNA vectors or chemical perturbants.[42,43] One recent study, for example, found that pVHL-defective cells are especially sensitive to agents that induce autophagy.[43] This finding is of special interest given the clinical activity of rapalogs, which likewise promote autophagy.

Germline mutations affecting succinate dehydrogenase (SDH) and fumarate hydratase (FH) have recently been linked to cancer and are also potentially linked to HIF deregulation.[44] The former have been linked to familial paragangliomas (including pheochromocytomas) and the latter to familial leiomyomatosis (cutaneous and uterine) and papillary renal carcinoma. SDH and FH mutations lead to the accumulation of succinate and fumarate, respectively, which interfere with the activities of 2-oxoglutarate–dependent dioxygenases, including the EglNs.[45–49] As a result, these mutations lead to inappropriate HIF activation and a state of "pseudohypoxia." Whether HIF is simply a marker of altered metabolism in these settings, or is an actual driver, is currently being explored. For example, indirect evidence, including genotype–phenotype correlations in VHL disease, argue that HIF deregulation does not play a causal role in pheochromocytoma.[16] Interestingly, mutations in isocitrate dehydrogenase 1 and 2 (IDH1 and IDH2) have been observed in some leukemias and brain tumors.[50–54] These mutations result in the production of 2-hydroxyglutarate, which is also suspected of altering 2-oxoglutarate-dependent enzyme activity.[55–57]

Enzymes are preferred targets in the pharmaceutical industry because they frequently contain clefts or pockets that can bind to drug-like small organic molecules. Indeed, many recently approved anticancer agents are small ATP-like molecules that inhibit particular kinases. The EglN prolyl hydroxylases belong to a large superfamily of iron and 2-oxoglutarate–dependent dioxygenases.[58] These enzymes can be inhibited with drug-like molecules that interfere with either iron or 2-oxoglutarate utilization. A further exploration of the biology of these enzymes therefore seems warranted.

EglN1 (PHD2) is being explored as a potential target for anemia, as outlined above. A recent study also found that haploinsufficiency for EglN1 suppressed tumor growth, apparently as a result of tumor vessel normalization.[59] Therefore, it is difficult to predict

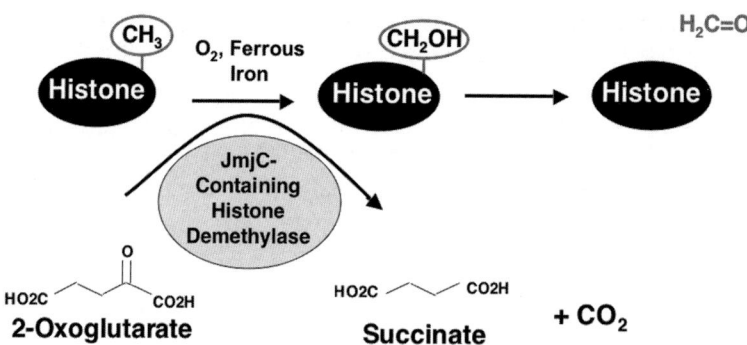

Figure 2. JmjC-histone demethylase activity. Hydroxylation of a histone methyl group by a JmjC domain-containing histone methylase leads to histone demethylation because the hydroxylated methyl group is unstable and spontaneously given off as formaldehyde.

whether EglN1 inhibitors will have protumorigenic or antitumorigenic effects *in vivo*.

EglN2 and EglN3 appear to have HIF-independent functions that might be relevant to tumor growth. EglN2 (PHD1) is transcriptionally induced when estrogen receptor positive breast cancer cells are induced to proliferate with estrogen.[60] We showed that EglN2, in a HIF-independent manner, indirectly controls Cyclin D1.[61] Cyclin D1 levels are diminished in *EglN2$^{-/-}$* cells and tissues including in lactating mammary glands, which display defects reminiscent of those seen in *Cyclin D1$^{-/-}$* glands.[62] Downregulation of EglN2, using shRNA technology, inhibits the proliferation of a variety of cancer cells, including breast cancer cells. This defect can be rescued by wild-type, but not catalytic-dead, EglN2 as well as by Cyclin D1 itself. These findings suggest that EglN2 inhibitors might have antitumor effects, especially in estrogen-dependent breast cancers.

EglN3 (PHD3) is induced when NGF is withdrawn from neurons and appears to be both necessary and sufficient to promote apoptosis in this setting.[63–66] EglN3 can also, at least when overproduced, induced apoptosis in a variety of cell types, in contrast to EglN1 and EglN2, and appears to do so in a HIF-independent manner.[67,68] How EglN3 induces apoptosis is incompletely understood but appears to involve KIF1Bβ, which is a candidate tumor suppressor located at 1p36.[67,69,70] Recent studies suggest that EglN3 agonists, such as 2-oxoglutarate mimetics, might be used to augment cancer cell apoptosis.[71,72]

A number of histone demethylases that share a JmjC domain were recently found to belong to the 2-oxoglutarate–dependent dioxygenase family[73,74] (Fig. 2). Interestingly, a number of these appear to be overexpressed or mutated in cancer, including JAR1DA, JARID1B, JARID1C, UTX, and GASC1.[37,75–80] JARID1A (also called RBP2 or KDM5A) was originally identified as cellular protein capable of binding to the retinoblastoma tumor suppressor protein (pRB).[81] pRB can induce an acute G1/S block, promote senescence, and/or promote differentiation when reintroduced into pRB-defective tumor cells. Tumor suppression by pRB is due, at least in part, to its ability to repress E2F-dependent promoters. Surprisingly, we found that certain pRB variants (natural and engineered) that cannot bind to E2F, and are incapable of repressing transcription, can nonetheless promote senescence and differentiation.[82] Such variants, however, preserve the ability to bind to JARID1A. Moreover, elimination of JARID1A, using either siRNA or genetically engineered cells, promotes senescence, differentiation, and loss of "stemness" in vitro[83] (Qin Yan and W.G.K., unpublished data). Conversely, a recent report suggested that increased expression of JARID1A mediates some forms of anticancer drug resistance by promoting a more stem cell-like phenotype.[84] Similarly, JARID1B promotes breast cancer growth *in vivo*[85] and appears to maintain a stem cell-like melanoma cell population.[86]

These considerations raise the possibility that changes in the levels of oxygen and specific metabolites (such as 2-oxoglutarate) will have protean biological effects through changes in the activities of various 2-oxoglutarate–dependent dioxygenases, including the enzymes dedicated to the regulation of HIF and chromatin structure. As a corollary, drugs that inhibit specific members of this family of enzymes might ultimately prove useful in the treatment of a variety of human diseases, including cancer.

Conflicts of interest

The authors declare no conflicts of interest.

References

1. Kaelin, W.G. 2002. Molecular basis of the VHL hereditary cancer syndrome. *Nat Rev Cancer.* **2:** 673–682.
2. Kaelin, W.G. Jr. & P.J. Ratcliffe. 2008. Oxygen sensing by metazoans: the central role of the HIF hydroxylase pathway. *Mol. Cell.* **30:** 393–402.
3. Hirsila, M. *et al.* 2003. Characterization of the human prolyl 4-hydroxylases that modify the hypoxia-inducible factor. *J. Biol. Chem.* **278:** 30772–30780.
4. McNeill, L.A. *et al.* 2002. The use of dioxygen by HIF prolyl hydroxylase (PHD1). *Bioorg. Med. Chem. Lett.* **12:** 1547–1550.
5. Berra, E. *et al.* 2003. HIF prolyl-hydroxylase 2 is the key oxygen sensor setting low steady-state levels of HIF-1alpha in normoxia. *Embo. J.* **22:** 4082–4090.
6. Appelhoff, R.J. *et al.* 2004. Differential function of the prolyl hydroxylases PHD1, PHD2, and PHD3 in the regulation of hypoxia-inducible factor. *J. Biol. Chem.* **279:** 38458–38465.
7. Minamishima, Y.A. *et al.* 2009. A feedback loop involving the Phd3 prolyl hydroxylase tunes the mammalian hypoxic response in vivo. *Mol. Cell. Biol.* **29:** 5729–5741.
8. Minamishima, Y.A. *et al.* 2008. Somatic inactivation of the PHD2 prolyl hydroxylase causes polycythemia and congestive heart failure. *Blood* **111:** 3236–3244.
9. Takeda, K. *et al.* 2008. Regulation of adult erythropoiesis by prolyl hydroxylase domain proteins. *Blood* **111:** 3229–3235.
10. Percy, M.J. *et al.* 2006. A family with erythrocytosis establishes a role for prolyl hydroxylase domain protein 2 in oxygen homeostasis. *Proc. Natl. Acad. Sci. USA* **103:** 654–659.
11. Percy, M.J. *et al.* 2007. A novel erythrocytosis-associated PHD2 mutation suggests the location of a HIF binding groove. *Blood* **110:** 2193–2196.
12. Dowling, T.C. 2007. Prevalence, etiology, and consequences of anemia and clinical and economic benefits of anemia correction in patients with chronic kidney disease: an overview. *Am. J. Health Syst. Pharm.* **64:** S3–7; quiz S23–25.
13. Minamishima, Y.A. & W.G. Kaelin Jr. Reactivation of hepatic EPO synthesis in mice after PHD loss. *Science* **329:** 407.
14. Safran, M. *et al.* 2006. Mouse model for noninvasive imaging of HIF prolyl hydroxylase activity: assessment of an oral agent that stimulates erythropoietin production. *Proc. Natl. Acad. Sci. USA* **103:** 105–110.
15. Kaelin, W.G., Jr. 2008. The von Hippel-Lindau tumour suppressor protein: O_2 sensing and cancer. *Nat. Rev. Cancer.* **8:** 865–873.
16. Kaelin, W.G., Jr. 2007. The von hippel-lindau tumor suppressor protein: an update. *Methods Enzymol.* **435:** 371–383.
17. Gordan, J.D. *et al.* 2007. HIF-2alpha promotes hypoxic cell proliferation by enhancing c-myc transcriptional activity. *Cancer Cell.* **11:** 335–347.
18. Gordan, J.D. *et al.* 2008. HIF-alpha effects on c-Myc distinguish two subtypes of sporadic VHL-deficient clear cell renal carcinoma. *Cancer Cell.* **14:** 435–446.
19. Maxwell, P. *et al.* 1999. The von Hippel-Lindau gene product is necessary for oxgyen-dependent proteolysis of hypoxia-inducible factor a subunits. *Nature* **399:** 271–275.
20. Kondo, K. *et al.* 2002. Inhibition of HIF is necessary for tumor suppression by the von Hippel-Lindau protein. *Cancer Cell.* **1:** 237–246.
21. Maranchie, J.K. *et al.* 2002. The contribution of VHL substrate binding and HIF1-alpha to the phenotype of VHL loss in renal cell carcinoma. *Cancer Cell.* **1:** 247–255.
22. Kondo, K. *et al.* 2003. Inhibition of HIF2alpha is sufficient to suppress pVHL-defective tumor growth. *PLos Biol.* **1:** 439–444.
23. Zimmer, M. *et al.* 2004. Inhibition of hypoxia-inducible factor is sufficient for growth suppression of VHL-/- tumors. *Mol. Cancer Res.* **2:** 89–95.
24. Kim, W.Y. *et al.* 2006. Failure to prolyl hydroxylate hypoxia-inducible factor alpha phenocopies VHL inactivation in vivo. *Embo J.* **25:** 4650–4662.
25. Rankin, E.B. *et al.* 2007. Hypoxia-inducible factor-2 (HIF-2) regulates hepatic erythropoietin in vivo. *J. Clin. Invest.* **117:** 1068–1077.
26. Rankin, E.B. *et al.* 2008. Hypoxia-inducible factor-2 regulates vascular tumorigenesis in mice. *Oncogene* **27:** 5354–5358.
27. Rankin, E.B. *et al.* 2009. HIF-2 regulates hepatic lipid metabolism. *Mol. Cel. Biol.* **29:** 4527–4538.
28. Mandriota, S.J. *et al.* 2002. HIF activation identifies early lesions in VHL kidneys: evidence for site-specific tumor suppressor function in the nephron. *Cancer Cell.* **1:** 459–468.
29. Escudier, B. *et al.* 2007. Bevacizumab plus interferon alfa-2a for treatment of metastatic renal cell carcinoma: a randomised, double-blind phase III trial. *Lancet* **370:** 2103–2111.
30. Escudier, B. *et al.* 2007. Sorafenib in advanced clear-cell renal-cell carcinoma. *N. Engl. J. Med.* **356:** 125–134.
31. Motzer, R.J. *et al.* 2007. Sunitinib versus interferon alfa in metastatic renal-cell carcinoma. *N. Engl. J. Med.* **356:** 115–124.
32. Sternberg, C.N. *et al.* Pazopanib in locally advanced or metastatic renal cell carcinoma: results of a randomized phase III trial. *J. Clin. Oncol.* **28:** 1061–1068.
33. Hudes, G. *et al.* 2006. A phase 3, randomized, 3-arm study of temsirolimus (TEMSR) or interferon-alpha (IFN) or the combination of TEMSR + IFN in the treatment of first-line, poor-risk *patients with advanced renal cell carcinoma (adv RCC). In JCO, 2006 ASCO Annual Meetings Proceedings Part I.* 24: LBA4.
34. Motzer, R.J. *et al.* 2008. Efficacy of everolimus in advanced renal cell carcinoma: a double-blind, randomised, placebo-controlled phase III trial. *Lancet* **372:** 449–456.
35. Guertin, D.A. & D.M. Sabatini. 2007. Defining the role of mTOR in cancer. *Cancer Cell.* **12:** 9–22.
36. Toschi, A. *et al.* 2008. Differential dependence of HIF1alpha and HIF2alpha on mTORC1 and mTORC2. *J. Biol. Chem.* **283:** 34495–34499.

37. Dalgliesh, G.L. *et al.* 2010. Systematic sequencing of renal carcinoma reveals inactivation of histone modifying genes. *Nature* **463:** 360–363.

38. Beroukhim, R. *et al.* 2009. Patterns of gene expression and copy-number alterations in von-hippel lindau disease-associated and sporadic clear cell carcinoma of the kidney. *Cancer Res.* **69:** 4674–4681.

39. Chen, M. *et al.* 2009. Genome-wide profiling of chromosomal alterations in renal cell carcinoma using high-density single nucleotide polymorphism arrays. *Int. J. Cancer* **125:** 2342–2348.

40. Yoshimoto, T. *et al.* 2007. High-resolution analysis of DNA copy number alterations and gene expression in renal clear cell carcinoma. *J. Pathol.* **213:** 392–401.

41. Cifola, I. *et al.* 2008. Genome-wide screening of copy number alterations and LOH events in renal cell carcinomas and integration with gene expression profile. *Mol. Cancer* **7:** 6.

42. Bommi-Reddy, A. *et al.* 2008. Kinase requirements in human cells: III. Altered kinase requirements in VHL-/- cancer cells detected in a pilot synthetic lethal screen. *Proc. Natl Acad. Sci. USA* **105:** 16484–16489.

43. Turcotte, S. *et al.* 2008. A molecule targeting VHL-deficient renal cell carcinoma that induces autophagy. *Cancer Cell.* **14:** 90–102.

44. Kaelin, W.G., Jr. 2009. SDH5 mutations and familial paraganglioma: somewhere Warburg is smiling. *Cancer Cell.* **16:** 180–182.

45. Koivunen, P. *et al.* 2007. Inhibition of hypoxia-inducible factor (HIF) hydroxylases by citric acid cycle intermediates: possible links between cell metabolism and stabilization of HIF. *J. Biol. Chem.* **282:** 4524–4532.

46. Pollard, P.J. *et al.* 2005. Accumulation of Krebs cycle intermediates and over-expression of HIF1alpha in tumours which result from germline FH and SDH mutations. *Hum. Mol. Genet.* **14:** 2231–2239.

47. Selak, M.A. *et al.* 2005. Succinate links TCA cycle dysfunction to oncogenesis by inhibiting HIF-alpha prolyl hydroxylase. *Cancer Cell.* **7:** 77–85.

48. Pollard, P.J. *et al.* 2007. Targeted inactivation of fh1 causes proliferative renal cyst development and activation of the hypoxia pathway. *Cancer Cell.* **11:** 311–319.

49. Dahia, P.L. *et al.* 2005. A HIF1alpha regulatory loop links hypoxia and mitochondrial signals in pheochromocytomas. *PLoS Genet* **1:** 72–80.

50. Balss, J. *et al.* 2008. Analysis of the IDH1 codon 132 mutation in brain tumors. *Acta Neuropathol.* **116:** 597–602.

51. Parsons, D.W. *et al.* 2008. An integrated genomic analysis of human glioblastoma multiforme. *Science* **321:** 1807–1812.

52. Watanabe, T. *et al.* 2009. IDH1 mutations are early events in the development of astrocytomas and oligodendrogliomas. *Am. J. Pathol.* **174:** 1149–1153.

53. Yan, H. *et al.* 2009. IDH1 and IDH2 mutations in gliomas. *N. Engl. J. Med.* **360:** 765–773.

54. Marcucci, G. *et al.* IDH1 and IDH2 gene mutations identify novel molecular subsets within de novo cytogenetically normal acute myeloid leukemia: a Cancer and Leukemia Group B study. *J. Clin. Oncol.* **28:** 2348–2355.

55. Ward, P.S. *et al.* 2010. The common feature of leukemia-associated IDH1 and IDH2 mutations is a neomorphic enzyme activity converting alpha-ketoglutarate to 2-hydroxyglutarate. *Cancer Cell.* **17:** 225–234.

56. Dang, L. *et al.* 2009. Cancer-associated IDH1 mutations produce 2-hydroxyglutarate. *Nature* **462:** 739–744.

57. Gross, S. *et al.* 2010. Cancer-associated metabolite 2-hydroxyglutarate accumulates in acute myelogenous leukemia with isocitrate dehydrogenase 1 and 2 mutations. *J. Exp. Med.* **207:** 339–344.

58. Aravind, L. & E.V. Koonin. 2001. The DNA-repair protein AlkB, EGL-9, and leprecan define new families of 2-oxoglutarate- and iron-dependent dioxygenases. *Genome Bio.* **2:** research0007.1–0007.8.

59. Mazzone, M. *et al.* 2009. Heterozygous deficiency of PHD2 restores tumor oxygenation and inhibits metastasis via endothelial normalization. *Cell* **136:** 839–851.

60. Seth, P. *et al.* 2002. Novel estrogen and tamoxifen induced genes identified by SAGE (Serial Analysis of Gene Expression). *Oncogene* **21:** 836–843.

61. Zhang, Q. *et al.* 2009. Control of cyclin D1 and breast tumorigenesis by the EglN2 prolyl hydroxylase. *Cancer Cell.* **16:** 413–424.

62. Sicinski, P. *et al.* 1995. Cyclin D1 provides a link between development and oncogenesis in the retina and breast. *Cell* **82:** 621–630.

63. Lee, S. *et al.* 2005. Neuronal apoptosis linked to EglN3 prolyl hydroxylase and familial pheochromocytoma genes: developmental culling and cancer. *Cancer Cell.* **8:** 155–167.

64. Lipscomb, E. *et al.* 1999. Expression of the SM-20 gene promotes death in nerve growth factor-dependent sympathetic neurons. *J. Neurochem.* **73:** 429–432.

65. Lipscomb, E. P. Sarmiere & R. Freeman. 2001. SM-20 is a novel mitochondrial protein that causes caspase-dependent cell death in nerve growth factor-dependent neurons. *J. Biol. Chem.* **276:** 11775–11782.

66. Bishop, T. *et al.* 2008. Abnormal sympathoadrenal development and systemic hypotension in PHD3-/- mice. *Mol. Cell. Biol.* **28:** 3386–3400.

67. Schlisio, S. *et al.* 2008. The kinesin KIF1Bbeta acts downstream from EglN3 to induce apoptosis and is a potential 1p36 tumor suppressor. *Genes Dev.* **22:** 884–893.

68. Rantanen, K. *et al.* 2008. Prolyl hydroxylase PHD3 activates oxygen-dependent protein aggregation. *Mol. Biol. Cell.* **19:** 2231–2240.

69. Yeh, I.T. *et al.* 2008. A germline mutation of the KIF1B beta gene on 1p36 in a family with neural and nonneural tumors. *Hum Genet.* **124:** 279–285.

70. Munirajan, A.K. *et al.* 2008. KIF1Bbeta functions as a haploinsufficient tumor suppressor gene mapped to chromosome 1p36.2 by inducing apoptotic cell death. *J. Biol. Chem.* **283:** 24426–24434.

71. MacKenzie, E.D. *et al.* 2007. Cell-permeating alpha-ketoglutarate derivatives alleviate pseudohypoxia in succinate dehydrogenase-deficient cells. *Mol. Cell Biol.* **27:** 3282–3289.

72. Tennant, D.A. *et al.* 2009. Reactivating HIF prolyl hydroxylases under hypoxia results in metabolic catastrophe and cell death. *Oncogene* **28:** 4009–4021.

73. Klose, R.J. E.M. Kallin & Y. Zhang. 2006. JmjC-domain-containing proteins and histone demethylation. *Nat. Rev. Genet.* **7:** 715–727.

74. Takeuchi, T. *et al.* 2006. Roles of jumonji and jumonji family genes in chromatin regulation and development. *Dev Dyn.* **235:** 2449–2459.

75. Cloos, P.A. *et al.* 2006. The putative oncogene GASC1 demethylates tri- and dimethylated lysine 9 on histone H3. *Nature* **442:** 307–311.

76. Northcott, P.A. *et al.* 2009. Multiple recurrent genetic events converge on control of histone lysine methylation in medulloblastoma. *Nat. Genet.* **41:** 465–472.

77. van Haaften, G. *et al.* 2009. Somatic mutations of the histone H3K27 demethylase gene UTX in human cancer. *Nat. Genet.* **41:** 521–523.

78. Wang, G.G. *et al.* 2009. Haematopoietic malignancies caused by dysregulation of a chromatin-binding PHD finger. *Nature* **459:** 847–851.

79. Barrett, A. *et al.* 2002. PLU-1 nuclear protein, which is up-regulated in breast cancer, shows restricted expression in normal human adult tissues: a new cancer/testis antigen? *Int. J. Cancer* **101:** 581–588.

80. van Zutven, L.J. *et al.* 2006. Identification of NUP98 abnormalities in acute leukemia: JARID1A (12p13) as a new partner gene. *Genes Chromosomes Cancer* **45:** 437–446.

81. Defeo-Jones, D. *et al.* 1991. Cloning of cDNAs for cellular proteins that bind to the retinoblastoma gene product. *Nature* **352:** 251–254.

82. Sellers, W.R. *et al.* 1998. Stable binding to E2F is not required for the retinoblastoma protein to activate transcription, promote differentiation, and suppress tumor cell growth. *Genes Dev.* **12:** 95–106.

83. Benevolenskaya, E.V. *et al.* 2005. Binding of pRB to the PHD protein RBP2 promotes cellular differentiation. *Mol. Cell* **18:** 623–635.

84. Sharma, S.V. *et al.* 2010. A chromatin-mediated reversible drug-tolerant state in cancer cell subpopulations. *Cell* **141:** 69–80.

85. Yamane, K. *et al.* 2007. PLU-1 is an H3K4 demethylase involved in transcriptional repression and breast cancer cell proliferation. *Mol. Cell* **25:** 801–812.

86. Roesch, A. *et al.* 2010. A temporarily distinct subpopulation of slow-cycling melanoma cells is required for continuous tumor growth. *Cell* **141:** 583–594.

Ann. N.Y. Acad. Sci. ISSN 0077-8923

ANNALS OF THE NEW YORK ACADEMY OF SCIENCES
Issue: *Toward Personalized Medicine for Cancer*

Role of BNIP3 in proliferation and hypoxia-induced autophagy: implications for personalized cancer therapies

Meghan B. Azad[1,2,3] and Spencer B. Gibson[1,2,3]

[1]Manitoba Institute of Cell Biology, University of Manitoba, Winnipeg, Canada. [2]CancerCare Manitoba, University of Manitoba, Winnipeg, Canada. [3]Department of Biochemistry and Medical Genetics, University of Manitoba, Winnipeg, Canada

Address for correspondence: Meghan B. Azad, ON5045-675 McDermot Ave., Winnipeg, Manitoba, Canada R3E 0V9. meghan.azad@hotmail.com

Autophagy is a regulated degradation pathway functioning in both cell survival and cell death. Its role in cancer is controversial because autophagy can be either protective or destructive to tumor cells, depending on individual genetic signatures and treatment conditions. Hypoxia is common in solid tumors, correlating with chemoresistance and poor prognosis. We have detected autophagic cell death in hypoxic cancer cells occurring independently of apoptosis through a mechanism involving the hypoxia-inducible protein, Bcl-2/E1B-nineteen kilodalton interacting protein (BNIP3). Loss of BNIP3 was protective against hypoxia-induced autophagy and cell death. Unexpectedly, BNIP3 ablation also caused differential cell cycle progression *in vitro* and increased cellularity *in vivo*. Collectively, these results support the emerging theory that autophagy could be effectively targeted as an alternative cell death pathway in hypoxic and/or apoptosis-resistant tumors. Furthermore, our data suggest that BNIP3 may be a potential target molecule in this pathway.

Keywords: autophagy; BNIP3; hypoxia; cancer; cell death; cancer therapy

Introduction: hypoxia and autophagy in cancer

Hypoxia is a driving factor in cancer progression, contributing to tumor aggression and poor prognosis.[1] Defective tumor vasculature limits the delivery of oxygen and nutrients, often causing necrosis in the interior regions of solid tumors where the microenvironment is anoxic. However, surrounding hypoxic tumor cells can adapt, survive, and proliferate by exploiting the induction of survival factors. The cellular response to hypoxia leads to sustained angiogenesis and genomic instability, contributing to further tumor cell transformation.[1] Tumor hypoxia additionally selects for gene mutations in regulators of cell proliferation, such as p53 and epidermal growth factor receptor (EGFR), thereby driving the evolution of hypoxic cancer cells toward increased malignancy.[2] Indeed, the extent of tumor hypoxia correlates with neoplastic aggression, resistance to therapy, and reduced patient survival.[1] It is therefore important to understand the cell death mechanisms involved (and evaded) during hypoxia in order to develop improved cancer treatment strategies.

Autophagy is the cellular pathway of "self digestion," a regulated lysosomal pathway for the degradation and recycling of long-lived proteins and organelles.[3] During autophagy, cytoplasmic constituents are sequestered into double-membraned autophagosomes, which are delivered to lysosomes and degraded. This process generates nucleotides, amino acids, and fatty acids, which are recycled for ATP generation and macromolecular synthesis. Autophagy is consistently active at low basal levels to maintain cellular homeostasis; however, it is also transiently upregulated as a survival response to various stress stimuli such as nutrient deprivation.[3] In addition, autophagy has the capacity to promote apoptosis or induce "autophagic cell death," the result of excessive self-digestion.[4] Several studies, including our own, have demonstrated both pro-survival and prodeath roles for hypoxia-induced autophagy in various contexts.[5] Additional research

doi: 10.1111/j.1749-6632.2010.05778.x

suggests that autophagy plays a significant role in cancer progression and could be a target for treatment.[6]

Because of its contradictory association with both survival and cell death, the role of autophagy in cancer is both complex and controversial.[6–8] Several studies point towards a cancer-promoting role for autophagy, whereas others support an anticancer role for the pathway. Accordingly, numerous reports assert the benefits of autophagy inhibition in cancer therapy, yet there is equally compelling evidence to contend autophagy induction as a therapeutic approach.

In support of autophagy as a procancer mechanism, it has been shown that tumor cells can exploit autophagy as a survival mechanism in the harsh tumor microenvironment, in order to sustain viability during periods of nutrient limitation, growth factor deprivation and metabolic stress.[9,10] For example, a recent study demonstrated that autophagy is required for survival and anchorage-independent growth of tumorigenic ductal carcinoma *in situ* (DCIS) cells, linking autophagy to breast cancer progression.[11] In contrast, other studies indicate that autophagy can function as a tumor suppression mechanism. Indeed, cancer cells often display a reduced autophagic capacity compared to their normal counterparts, suggesting that defective autophagy may play a role in malignant transformation.[12] In support of this theory, the autophagy gene *Beclin-1* has been identified as a haploinsufficient tumor suppressor in mice, and was shown to be monoallelically deleted in 40–75% of sporadic human breast, ovarian, and prostate tumors.[13,14] The mechanism by which autophagy inhibits tumorigenesis is unclear, but it may involve "mitochondrial quality control": prevention of oxidative damage and mutagenesis through the removal of damaged mitochondria, which are a major source of toxic reactive oxygen species.[6] Recent evidence indicates that autophagy may also suppress tumorigenesis through specific elimination of p62, an adaptor protein that promotes oxidative stress, genome damage, and tumorigenesis upon accumulation.[15]

As outlined above, autophagy can have entirely opposite consequences for tumor cells depending on the circumstances: survival and tumorigenesis, or cell death and tumor suppression. Accordingly, there is intense debate and conflicting evidence surrounding the role of autophagy in cancer therapy.[5,16,17] Many anticancer agents induce autophagy; however, it remains questionable whether the observed autophagic response is a survival attempt by tumor cells, or a killing mechanism of anticancer agents. For instance, studies have demonstrated the induction of autophagy by cancer cells as a protective response to several therapies, including: tamoxifen, cisplatin, perifosine, the HDAC inhibitor SAHA, the proteasome inhibitor MG-132, and the BH3-mimetic GX15-070.[18–20] Many of these agents exhibit increased cytotoxicity when autophagy is inhibited, prompting clinical trials to test the therapeutic efficacy of combining autophagy inhibitors with existing anticancer drugs.[17] On the contrary, autophagy has been shown to enhance or directly mediate the cytotoxicity of other cancer therapies including acadesine/AICAR, resveratrol, valproic acid, arsenic trioxide, temozolomide, endostatin, and imiquimod.[18,21,22] Conflicting reports indicate that radiation toxicity may be enhanced or inhibited by autophagy in different tumors, suggesting that further research is required before manipulation of autophagy can be clinically applied as a radio-sensitizing strategy.[23,24] Nevertheless, given that many tumors are characterized by defects in apoptosis, induction of autophagic cell death by chemotherapy or radiation represents a promising alternative therapeutic approach.[25]

In summary, autophagy is intricately involved in both tumorigenesis and the hypoxic response, representing an attractive new target for cancer therapy. Current data suggests that, depending on individual tumor characteristics and treatment regimens, either the induction or the inhibition of autophagy may provide therapeutic benefit for patients. Further studies are required to establish the precise role of autophagy during malignant transformation and tumor progression, which may ultimately lead to new therapeutic strategies in cancer.

Hypoxic cancer cells can undergo autophagic cell death independently of apoptosis

Although cells deprived of oxygen will initially employ adaptive and survival strategies, severe or sustained hypoxia ultimately leads to cell death. The precise mechanisms of hypoxia-induced cell death remain unclear as apoptosis, necrosis, and autophagy have all been reported in response to

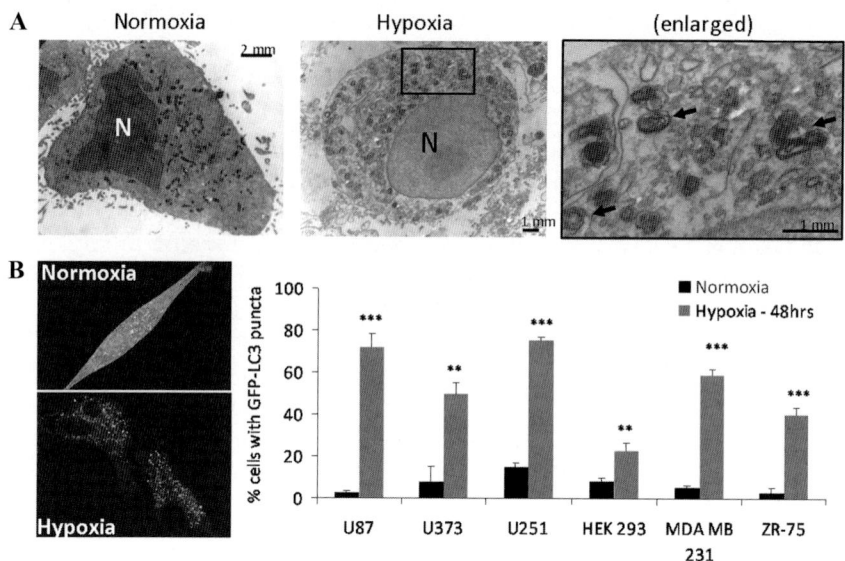

Figure 1. Hypoxia induces autophagy in multiple human cancer cell lines. (A) Electron microscopy: U87 cells were incubated in normoxia or hypoxia for 24 h followed by ultrastructural analysis by electron microscopy. Arrows indicate double-membraned autophagic vacuoles. (B) GFP–LC3 puncta: cells transiently expressing GFP–LC3 were incubated in normoxia or hypoxia for 24 h. GFP–LC3 displayed diffuse intracellular localization under normoxic conditions, whereas membrane translocation (punctate localization) indicative of autophagy was observed in hypoxic cells. Images were obtained using identical microscope settings, exposure times, and manipulations for brightness and contrast. The presence of GFP–LC3 puncta was quantified in transiently transfected normoxic and hypoxic cells. Two hundred cells per sample were counted for punctate versus diffuse staining (representative of three independent experiments). Error bars indicate standard deviation, and statistical analysis was by an unpaired student's t-test: $**P < 0.01, ***P < 0.001$. (Some of these data were previously published in Azad et al.[29])

hypoxic stress.[9,26,27] Autophagy is best characterized as a response to nutrient deprivation, an energy-limiting cellular stress.[28] Previously, "metabolic stress" (hypoxia combined with nutrient deprivation) has been shown to induce autophagy.[9] We recently published a series of experiments demonstrating that hypoxia alone can also induce autophagy, independent of apoptosis.[29]

We exposed several human cancer cell lines to prolonged hypoxia ($< 1\% \ O_2$, 24–72 h) and found that autophagy was universally induced, and cell death occurred after 48–72 h. Electron microscopy was used to identify double-membraned autophagosomes and localization of green fluorescent protein-tagged microtubule associated protein 1 light chain 3 (GFP-LC3, which is incorporated into autophagosome membranes) was also assessed (Fig. 1).[29] Interestingly, we found that hypoxia-induced autophagy contributed to cell death in some cell lines, but not in others (Fig. 2). This was determined using specific inhibitors for autophagy (3-methyladenine, 3-MA) and apoptosis (caspase inhibitor z-VAD-fmk). Whereas 3-MA was protective

against hypoxia-induced cell death in U87, U373, HEK293, ZR-75, and MDA-MB-231 cells, there was no protection afforded to U251 and MDA-MB-231-M cells. The reverse was true for z-VAD-fmk, which was protective in the latter two cell lines. Thus, although some cell lines induced autophagic cell death in hypoxia, others induced apoptosis. Notably, this differential induction of cell death pathways was not due to an inherent defect in apoptosis, because all cell lines were competent for etoposide-induced apoptosis as measured by caspase activation, cytochrome c release, and nuclear condensation.[29]

Taken together, these results show that hypoxic cancer cells can undergo autophagic cell death independent of apoptosis. In addition, hypoxia fails to induce apoptosis in multiple apoptosis-competent cell lines (U87, U373, HEK293, ZR-75, and MDA-MB-231), yet successfully triggers apoptosis in others (U251 and MDA-MB-231-M). The mechanism for the preference between autophagy and apoptosis under hypoxia in specific cells is currently unknown, and will be the focus of future investigations. Nevertheless, these are significant findings,

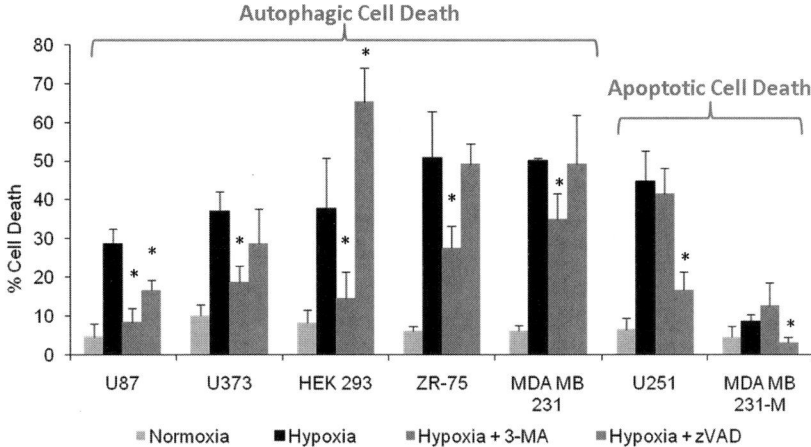

Figure 2. Hypoxia differentially induces apoptosis or autophagic cell death in different cancer cell lines. Cells were incubated in hypoxia for 48 h in the presence or absence of the autophagy inhibitor 3-MA, or the apoptosis inhibitor z-VAD-fmk. Total cell death was determined by membrane permeability assay. For cell lines where 3-MA was protective, hypoxia-induced cell death was classified as autophagic. For cell lines where z-VAD-fmk was protective, hypoxia-induced cell death was classified as apoptotic. All results represent three independent experiments, and error bars indicate the standard deviation. Statistical analysis was by an unpaired t-test: $^*P < 0.05$, $^{**}P < 0.01$ (relative to hypoxia alone for each cell line).

which contribute to the understanding of cell death mechanisms in hypoxia, and provide evidence for physiologically relevant autophagic cell death in apoptosis-competent cells. Furthermore, this research supports the hypothesis that targeting autophagy as an alternative cell death pathway may lead to promising new cancer treatment strategies.

BNIP3 plays a pivotal role in hypoxia-induced autophagic cell death

In order to successfully target autophagic cell death as a cancer treatment strategy, individual target molecules must be identified. Ubiquitous autophagy proteins are not ideal targets because autophagy is a critical pathway for homeostasis in normal cells.[30] We hypothesize that Bcl-2/E1B-nineteen kilodalton interacting protein (BNIP3) may represent a more "cancer-specific" autophagy target molecule because it is selectively induced during hypoxia, which is characteristic of solid tumors. Furthermore, we have recently shown that BNIP3 plays a pivotal role in the hypoxia-induced autophagic death of cancer cells.[29,31]

BNIP3 is a prodeath Bcl-2 family member that is upregulated under hypoxic conditions.[32] In transformed and cancer cells, forced overexpression of BNIP3 induces "nonapoptotic" cell death that is characterized by localization to the mitochondria, opening of the permeability transition pore, loss

of membrane potential and reactive oxygen species production.[32] In these cells, BNIP3-induced cell death is independent of caspase activation and cytochrome c release from the mitochondria. BNIP3 has been separately implicated in both autophagy and hypoxia-induced cell death.[31,33] In addition, BNIP3 has been implicated in cancer progression as it is silenced or mislocalized to the nucleus in some tumors.[32]

Similar to autophagy, BNIP3 has been described as prodeath in some instances, and prosurvival in others. For example, BNIP3 mediates both ceramide- and arsenic trioxide-induced autophagic cell death in cancer cells,[34,35] yet BNIP3-mediated "mitophagy" (selective autophagy of damaged mitochondria) is essential for mouse embryonic fibroblast survival in hypoxia.[36] In contrast, we have shown that BNIP3 plays a pivotal role in the hypoxia-induced autophagic cell death of cancer cells, as described below.[29]

Our recent work confirmed that BNIP3 mRNA and protein levels are elevated in HEK293, U87, and U251 cells at 48 and 72 h hypoxia (Fig. 3A), time points that correspond with increased cell death (Fig. 2). BNIP3 over-expression in normoxic cells induced a dramatic autophagic response, with GFP–LC3 puncta increasing from 2–3% in controls to 56–81% in BNIP3-transfected cells (Fig. 3B). Notably, deletion of the transmembrane domain

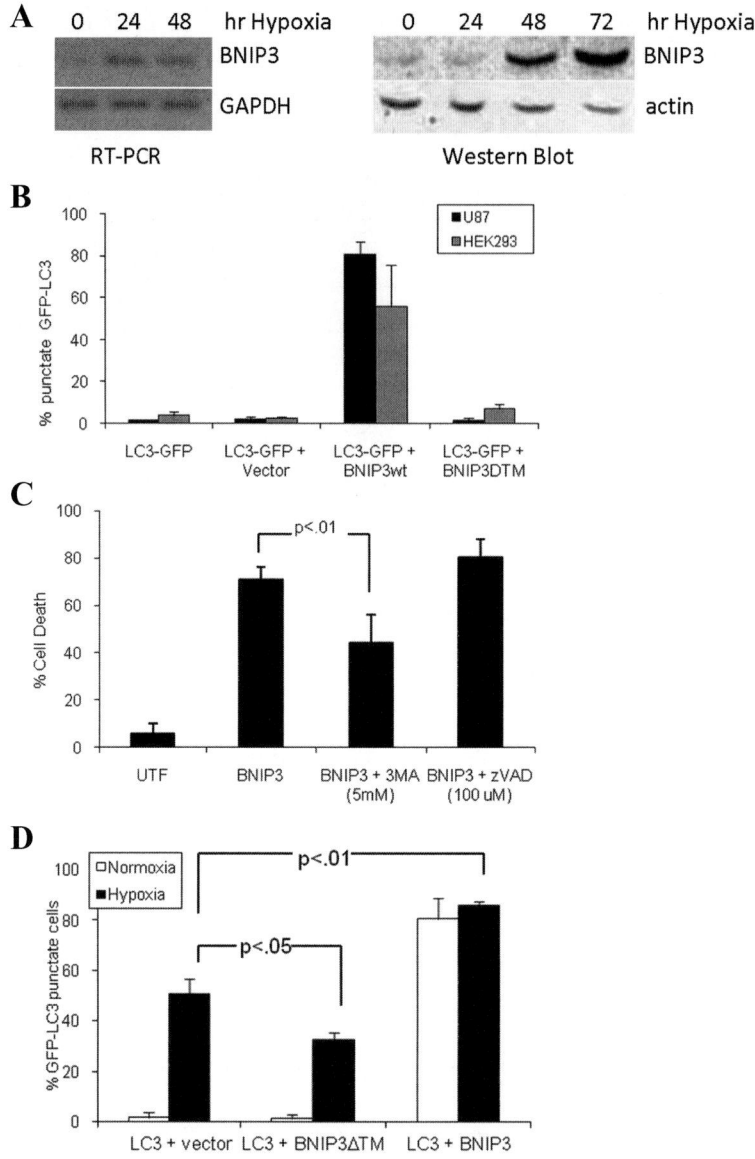

Figure 3. BNIP3 plays a pivotal role in hypoxia-induced autophagic cell death. (A) Hypoxia-induced BNIP3 expression: RT–PCR and Western blot analysis of BNIP3 expression in U87 cells cultured in normoxia or hypoxia for up to 72 h, with GAPDH or actin as a loading control. (B) BNIP3-induced autophagy: HEK293 and U87 cells were transiently transfected with the autophagy marker GFP–LC3, alone or with pcDNA3 (empty vector) or pcDNA3-BNIP3 or pcDNA3-BNIP3ΔTM. GFP–LC3 distribution (in cotransfected cells only) was assessed and quantified. Error bars indicate standard deviation of three independent experiments. (C) BNIP3-induced cell death: HEK293 cells were untransfected (control) or transfected with BNIP3. Cells were untreated or treated with 3-MA (5 mM) or z-VAD-fmk (100 μM) for 24 h posttransfection. Immunofluorescence for BNIP3 was performed, and cell death in BNIP3-positive cells was determined by assessing nuclear morphology. Error bars indicate standard deviation of three independent experiments. Statistical significance was determined by a two-tailed t-test. (D) HEK293 cells were transfected with GFP–LC3 plus empty vector, BNIP3 or BNIP3ΔTM, and incubated in normoxia or hypoxia for 24-h posttransfection. GFP–LC3 distribution (in cotransfected cells only) was assessed and quantified. (Some of these data were previously published in Azad et al.[29])

(which targets BNIP3 to mitochondria) completely abrogated BNIP3-induced autophagy. As expected, BNIP3 over-expression also induced cell death. We found that BNIP3-induced cell death was reduced by the autophagy inhibitor 3-MA (from 71% to 45%), but was unchanged by the caspase inhibitor z-VAD-fmk (Fig. 3C). Thus, our results suggest that in the cell lines tested, BNIP3-induced cell death is autophagic and not apoptotic.[29]

Previous studies have suggested that BNIP3 mediates hypoxia-induced cell death, because expression of the dominant-negative BNIP3ΔTM mutant or knock-down of the BNIP3 gene are protective in hypoxia.[31] We have now confirmed these findings using primary BNIP3[−/−] cells, which exhibit resistance to hypoxia compared to their wild-type counterparts (unpublished). Our work has further determined that, similar to hypoxia-induced cell death, hypoxia-induced autophagy is also reduced by BNIP3ΔTM or by BNIP3 knock-down, whereas it is enhanced by over-expression of wild-type BNIP3: GFP–LC3 puncta at 24 h hypoxia were observed in 53% of empty vector cells, which was reduced to 34% in BNIP3ΔTM-expressing cells, and increased to 86% for BNIP3-overexpressing cells (Fig. 3D).[29]

Collectively, these findings identify BNIP3 as an important mediator of hypoxia-induced autophagic cell death. Because it does not regulate basal autophagy, BNIP3 could theoretically be targeted to manipulate autophagy in hypoxic cancer cells without interrupting homeostasis in normal cells. Further research will be required to elucidate the mechanism of BNIP3-mediated autophagy in hypoxic cancer cells, and to establish methods of targeting BNIP3 in this pathway for therapeutic benefit.

A novel role for BNIP3 in cell cycle control and brain development?

Before BNIP3 can be rationally targeted for cancer therapy, its functional role must be fully defined. Ongoing studies in our laboratory suggest that BNIP3 may function outside of cell death and autophagy signaling, with additional roles in cell cycle control and development.

We ultimately intend to study hypoxia-related pathologies in BNIP3-null mice, in order to determine how BNIP3 contributes to disease processes such as tumorigenesis and ischemic injury. In preparation for these experiments, we have devoted considerable effort to determining whether any relevant baseline differences exist between BNIP3-null mice and their wild-type counterparts. Because BNIP3 has previously been implicated in the pathophysiology of brain tumors, neurodegeneration, and ischemic stroke,[32] our initial investigations have aimed to characterize the effect of BNIP3 ablation in the mouse brain.

Currently, little is known about the role of BNIP3 in normal brain function and development. The BNIP3-null mouse model has not yet been extensively studied, and research thus far has focused exclusively on the cardiovascular system.[37] However, limited evidence from wild-type studies has implicated BNIP3 in oligodendrocyte differentiation and developmental apoptosis in the postnatal rat brain.[38,39] In addition, hypoxia and hypoxia-inducible factor 1 (HIF-1) are established mediators of embryogenesis, and controlled cell death is an important aspect of mammalian development.[40] Accordingly, as a HIF-1 target gene and cell death mediator, BNIP3 is a likely candidate for the regulation of hypoxia-driven developmental processes. As discussed below, our unpublished data support this hypothesis.

In agreement with others,[37] we have found that homozygous BNIP3-null mice are born from heterozygous crosses at normal Mendelian ratios and show no increase in mortality or apparent physical abnormalities. Also in agreement with previous studies,[39,33] we have detected moderate BNIP3 expression in unstressed wild-type mouse brain and cultured astrocytes, suggesting that BNIP3 may play a functional role in brain physiology and development.

Our initial experiments in this area show that BNIP3 ablation in the developing mouse brain appears to cause increased cellularity, which persists into adulthood (work in progress). Although these findings support the hypothesis that BNIP3 mediates cell death (as opposed to mitophagy-dependent cell survival) during development, it remains possible that additional mechanisms are involved. Future studies will aim to define the mechanism, composition, and functional significance of increased cellularity in the BNIP3-null brain.

The observed increase in brain cellularity after BNIP3 ablation *in vivo* could be the result of increased cell proliferation, increased cell survival, and/or reduced cell death during development.

Indeed, we have found that loss of BNIP3 leads to reduced hypoxia-induced cell death in embryonic fibroblasts and astrocytes *in vitro* (unpublished). Again, our initial results indicate that BNIP3$^{-/-}$ astrocytes have a decreased rate of DNA replication and may also progress more slowly through the G2/M phase of cell division; however, further research is required to determine the impact of these differences on cell proliferation both *in vitro* and *in vivo*.

These initial results identify a potentially novel role for BNIP3 in the regulation of cell cycle progression and mammalian brain development. Although it has been widely studied as a mediator of cell death,[32] BNIP3 has never before been implicated in cell growth or proliferation. Further studies are required to fully elucidate the role of BNIP3 in proliferation *in vivo* and in different cell types, and to determine how BNIP3 may regulate DNA replication or promote cell division.

Discussion

Our research contributes to a growing body of evidence that implicates hypoxia-induced autophagy in multiple pathophysiological conditions including cancer, through both protective and destructive mechanisms.[5] The apparently contradictory functions for autophagy in hypoxia could be explained by a time-dependent "dual role" for autophagy in cell survival and cell death: early induction of autophagy may contribute to a protective response, whereas prolonged autophagy could lead to cell death. Indeed, we have found that autophagy is strongly induced in viable cells as quickly as 1 h following acute hypoxia (not shown). Because this rapid onset of autophagy occurs nearly 24 h before cell death is detectable, it likely serves as an initial survival strategy. Thus, our results are consistent with a model whereby rapidly induced autophagy could initially offer protection against hypoxic stress, whereas prolonged autophagy in hypoxia functions as a distinct mechanism of cell death, independently of apoptosis.

The two-faced role of autophagy in cancer presents an interesting therapeutic dilemma: should autophagy be induced, or inhibited during cancer treatment? Evidence exists to support both strategies, because many anticancer therapies induce protective autophagy (which can be inhibited to improve therapeutic efficacy), whereas other thera-

pies induce destructive autophagy (which enhances or directly mediates cytotoxicity). The role of autophagy in specific cancer therapies is discussed in several recent reviews.[4,17,18] Despite the dual role of autophagy in cancer cell survival and cell death, there is a consensus that autophagy should be considered as a new target for anticancer therapy. Our research provides strong evidence for this approach, identifying autophagy as a distinct mechanism of cell death in hypoxic cancer cells. The challenge going forward will be to determine when to stimulate, and when to inhibit autophagy for therapeutic benefit, based on treatment-specific anticancer mechanisms and individual tumor characteristics, such as stage of malignancy and apoptotic/autophagic capacity.

Together with previous studies, our research suggests that BNIP3 may be an important therapeutic target in the autophagy pathway. In theory, BNIP3 could be safely targeted without adverse effects because it is preferentially expressed during hypoxic stress, which is characteristic of tumors but not normal tissues. Further research will be required to elucidate the mechanism of BNIP3-mediated autophagy in hypoxic cancer cells, and to establish methods of targeting BNIP3 in this pathway for therapeutic benefit.

Our initial work also provides supportive evidence for BNIP3's role in brain development, and further identifies a related and potentially novel role for BNIP3 in the regulation of cell cycle progression. Although previous studies have suggested that BNIP3 is involved in development through its established cytoplasmic role in cell death,[38,39] our preliminary results indicate that BNIP3 may additionally regulate cell growth and proliferation (work in progress). Further research is required to confirm these findings, and to characterize the mechanisms involved. Beacuse BNIP3 has been observed in the nuclei of cultured human astrocytes,[33] it will be especially important to address the role of nuclear BNIP3 in brain development. Indeed, research from our lab has recently established that BNIP3 can bind directly to DNA and regulate gene expression.[32,33] Future studies will aim to determine how the absence of both nuclear and cytoplasmic BNIP3 contribute to the observed changes in cell proliferation and brain cellularity in BNIP3-null mice. Besides providing new insights into mammalian development, this research may ultimately have therapeutic implications if BNIP3-mediated proliferative pathways are found to play a role in BNIP3-related pathologies such as ischemic injury or cancer.

Taken together, our research advances the current understanding of autophagy signaling and its role in hypoxia, cell death, and cancer progression—concepts which are highly controversial at present. In addition, our work contributes to the body of knowledge surrounding the complex function of BNIP3, a cell death mediator with additional roles in autophagy, cancer, and development. We anticipate that comprehensive characterization of autophagy and BNIP3 will ultimately identify new targets for cancer therapy. Our work also highlights the importance of considering individual tumor characteristics (such as hypoxia, apoptotic and autophagic capacity, and BNIP3 status) during the design and delivery of cancer therapies.

Conflicts of interest

The authors declare no conflicts of interest.

References

1. Vaupel, P. 2004. The role of hypoxia-induced factors in tumor progression. *Oncologist* **9**(Suppl 5): 10–17.
2. Knisely, J.P. & S. Rockwell. 2002. Importance of hypoxia in the biology and treatment of brain tumors. *Neuroimaging Clin. N. Am.* **12**: 525–536.
3. Levine, B. 2005. Eating oneself and uninvited guests: autophagy-related pathways in cellular defense. *Cell* **120**: 159–162.
4. Coates, J.M., J.M. Galante & R.J. Bold. 2009. Cancer therapy beyond apoptosis: autophagy and anoikis as mechanisms of cell death. *J. Surg. Res.* [Epub ahead of print].
5. Mazure, N.M. & J. Pouyssegur. 2010. Hypoxia-induced autophagy: cell death or cell survival? *Curr. Opin. Cell Biol.* **22**: 177–180.
6. Jin, S. & E. White. 2007. Role of autophagy in cancer: management of metabolic stress. *Autophagy* **3**: 28–31.
7. Hippert, M.M., P.S. O'toole & A. Thorburn. 2006. Autophagy in cancer: good, bad, or both? *Cancer Res.* **66**: 9349–9351.
8. Azad, M.B., Y. Chen & S.B. Gibson. 2009. Regulation of autophagy by reactive oxygen species (ROS): implications for cancer progression and treatment. *Antioxid. Redox Signal.* **11**: 777–790.
9. Degenhardt, K., R. Mathew, B. Beaudoin, et al. 2006. Autophagy promotes tumor cell survival and restricts necrosis, inflammation, and tumorigenesis. *Cancer Cell* **10**: 51–64.
10. Lum, J.J., D.E. Bauer, M. Kong, et al. 2005. Growth factor regulation of autophagy and cell survival in the absence of apoptosis. *Cell* **120**: 237–248.
11. Espina, V., B.D. Mariani, R.I. Gallagher, et al. 2010. Malignant precursor cells pre-exist in human breast DCIS and require autophagy for survival. *PLoS One* **5**: e10240.
12. Qu, X., J. Yu, G. Bhagat, et al. 2003. Promotion of tumorigenesis by heterozygous disruption of the beclin 1 autophagy gene. *J. Clin. Invest.* **112**: 1809–1820.
13. Yue, Z., S. Jin, C. Yang, et al. 2003. Beclin 1, an autophagy gene essential for early embryonic development, is a haploinsufficient tumor suppressor. *Proc. Natl. Acad. Sci. USA* **100**: 15077–15082.
14. Liang, X.H., S. Jackson, M. Seaman, et al. 1999. Induction of autophagy and inhibition of tumorigenesis by beclin 1. *Nature* **402**: 672–676.
15. Mathew, R., C.M. Karp, B. Beaudoin, et al. 2009. Autophagy suppresses tumorigenesis through elimination of p62. *Cell* **137**: 1062–1075.
16. Dalby, K.N., I. Tekedereli, G. Lopez-Berestein & B. Ozpolat. 2010. Targeting the prodeath and prosurvival functions of autophagy as novel therapeutic strategies in cancer. *Autophagy* **6**: 322–329.
17. White, E. & R.S. DiPaola. 2009. The double-edged sword of autophagy modulation in cancer. *Clin. Cancer Res.* **15**: 5308–5316.
18. Kondo, Y. & S. Kondo. 2006. Autophagy and cancer therapy. *Autophagy* **2**: 85–90.
19. Pan, J., C. Cheng, S. Verstovsek, et al. 2010. The BH3-mimetic GX15-070 induces autophagy, potentiates the cytotoxicity of carboplatin and 5-fluorouracil in esophageal carcinoma cells. *Cancer Lett.* **293**: 167–174.
20. Wu, W.K., C.H. Cho, C.W. Lee, et al. 2010. Macroautophagy and ERK phosphorylation counteract the antiproliferative effect of proteasome inhibitor in gastric cancer cells. *Autophagy* **6**: 228–238.
21. Robert, G., I. Ben Sahra, A. Puissant, et al. 2009. Acadesine kills chronic myelogenous leukemia (CML) cells through PKC-dependent induction of autophagic cell death. *PLoS One* **4**: e7889.
22. Huang, S.W., K.T. Liu, C.C. Chang, et al. 2010. Imiquimod simultaneously induces autophagy and apoptosis in human basal cell carcinoma cells. *Br. J. Dermatol.* **163**: 310–320.
23. Zois, C.E. & M.I. Koukourakis. 2009. Radiation-induced autophagy in normal and cancer cells: towards novel cytoprotection and radio-sensitization policies? *Autophagy* **5**: 442–450.
24. Kim, K.W., L. Moretti, L.R. Mitchell, et al. 2010. Endoplasmic reticulum stress mediates radiation-induced autophagy by perk-eIF2alpha in caspase-3/7-deficient cells. *Oncogene* **29**: 3241–3251.
25. Lefranc, F., V. Facchini & R. Kiss. 2007. Proautophagic drugs: a novel means to combat apoptosis-resistant cancers, with a special emphasis on glioblastomas. *Oncologist* **12**: 1395–1403.
26. Brunelle, J.K. & N.S. Chandel. 2002. Oxygen deprivation induced cell death: an update. *Apoptosis* **7**: 475–482.
27. Hamacher-Brady, A., N.R. Brady & R.A. Gottlieb. 2006. Enhancing macroautophagy protects against ischemia/reperfusion injury in cardiac myocytes. *J. Biol. Chem.* **281**: 29776–29787.
28. Mizushima, N., A. Yamamoto, M. Matsui, et al. 2004. *In vivo* analysis of autophagy in response to nutrient starvation

using transgenic mice expressing a fluorescent autophago-some marker. *Mol. Biol. Cell* **15:** 1101–1111.

29. Azad, M.B., Y. Chen, E.S. Henson, *et al.* 2008. Hypoxia induces autophagic cell death in apoptosis-competent cells through a mechanism involving BNIP3. *Autophagy* **4:** 195–204.

30. Levine, B. & D.J. Klionsky. 2004. Development by self-digestion: molecular mechanisms and biological functions of autophagy. *Dev. Cell* **6:** 463–477.

31. Kothari, S., J. Cizeau, E. McMillan-Ward, *et al.* 2003. BNIP3 plays a role in hypoxic cell death in human epithelial cells that is inhibited by growth factors EGF and IGF. *Oncogene* **22:** 4734–4744.

32. Burton, T.R. & S.B. Gibson. 2009. The role of Bcl-2 family member BNIP3 in cell death and disease: NIPping at the heels of cell death. *Cell Death Differ.* **16:** 515–523.

33. Burton, T.R., E.S. Henson, P. Baijal, *et al.* 2006. The pro-cell death Bcl-2 family member, BNIP3, is localized to the nucleus of human glial cells: implications for glioblastoma multiforme tumor cell survival under hypoxia. *Int. J. Cancer* **118:** 1660–1669.

34. Kanzawa, T., L. Zhang, L. Xiao, *et al.* 2005. Arsenic trioxide induces autophagic cell death in malignant glioma cells by upregulation of mitochondrial cell death protein BNIP3. *Oncogene* **24:** 980–991.

35. Daido, S., T. Kanzawa, A. Yamamoto, *et al.* 2004. Pivotal role of the cell death factor BNIP3 in ceramide-induced autophagic cell death in malignant glioma cells. *Cancer Res.* **64:** 4286–4293.

36. Zhang, H., M. Bosch-Marce, L.A. Shimoda, *et al.* 2008. Mitochondrial autophagy is an HIF-1-dependent adaptive metabolic response to hypoxia. *J. Biol. Chem.* **283:** 10892–10903.

37. Diwan, A., M. Krenz, F.M. Syed, *et al.* 2007. Inhibition of ischemic cardiomyocyte apoptosis through targeted ablation of Bnip3 restrains postinfarction remodeling in mice. *J. Clin. Invest.* **117:** 2825–2833.

38. Itoh, T., A. Itoh & D. Pleasure. 2003. Bcl-2-related protein family gene expression during oligodendroglial differentiation. *J. Neurochem.* **85:** 1500–1512.

39. Sandau, U.S. & R.J. Handa. 2006. Localization and developmental ontogeny of the pro-apoptotic Bnip3 mRNA in the postnatal rat cortex and hippocampus. *Brain Res.* **1100:** 55–63.

40. Dunwoodie, S.L. 2009. The role of hypoxia in development of the Mammalian embryo. *Dev. Cell* **17:** 755–773.

Ann. N.Y. Acad. Sci. ISSN 0077-8923

ANNALS OF THE NEW YORK ACADEMY OF SCIENCES

Issue: *Toward Personalized Medicine for Cancer*

Discovery of genomic alterations through coregulation analysis of closely linked genes: a frequent gain in 17q25.3 in prostate cancer

Raquel Bermudo,[1,2] David Abia,[3] Daniel Benitez,[4,*] Anna Carrió,[5] Ramon Vilella,[4] Ángel R. Ortiz,[3,‡] Timothy M. Thomson,[1,†] and Pedro L. Fernández[2,5,†]

[1]Department of Cell Biology, Instituto de Biología Molecular de Barcelona, Consejo Superior de Investigaciones Científicas, Barcelona, Spain. [2]Institut d'Investigacions Biomèdiques August Pi i Sunyer, Barcelona, Spain. [3]Bioinformatics Unit, Centro de Biología Molecular Severo Ochoa, Consejo Superior de Investigaciones Científicas and Universidad Autónoma de Madrid, Cantoblanco, Madrid, Spain. [4]Departments of Immunology, Hospital Clínic de Barcelona, Barcelona, Spain. [5]Pathology, Hospital Clínic de Barcelona, Barcelona, Spain

Addresses for correspondence: Pedro L. Fernández, M.D., Ph.D., Department of Pathology, Hospital Clínic de Barcelona, c. Villarroel 170, 08036 Barcelona, Spain. plfernan@clinic.ub.es. Timothy M. Thomson, M.D., Ph.D., Department of Cell Biology, Instituto de Biología Molecular de Barcelona, Barcelona Science Park, Helix Building, Room 02A20, c. Baldiri Reixac 15-21, 08028 Barcelona, Spain. titbmc@ibmb.csic.es

Despite its high incidence as the second most common tumor in males worldwide, primary prostate cancer has been associated with few recurrent chromosomal gains and deletions that are consistent across various studies. Few studies have explored how chromosomal alterations are coupled to abnormal gene expression. Here, we review the major genomic aberrations associated with prostate cancer and describe how detailed transcriptional and computational analyses allowed us to discover a recurrent chromosomal gain in a small region on chromosome 17. Fluorescent *in situ* hybridization confirmed the presence of a copy number gain in 17q25.3 in tumor-associated preneoplastic lesions of the prostate, 65% of primary tumors, and metastatic samples. These results suggest the involvement of this gain at all steps of prostate cancer progression.

Keywords: prostate cancer; copy number alterations; transcriptional profiling; 17q25.3

Chromosomal alterations in prostate cancer

Classical cytogenetic studies and, more recently, high-throughput genomic studies, have unveiled many chromosomal alterations associated with prostate cancer (PCa), the second most frequent tumor in males worldwide.[1]

Both clinically and histopathologically, PCa is a highly heterogeneous disease. At the histological level, PCa is usually found as a complex mixture of benign tissue, multiple neoplastic foci with distinct molecular alterations, and foci of the preneoplastic lesion prostate intraepithelial neoplasia (PIN). A study, based on genome-wide studies, shows that the general pattern of chromosomal losses and gains displays many similarities between PIN lesions and tumors. This occurs despite the fact that tumors present a significantly a higher number of abnormalities.[2] Interestingly, in both lesions, losses are more frequent than gains, which suggests that haploinsufficiency in one or more genes may underlie the initial steps of prostate carcinogenesis.[2]

One of the most recurrent gains in primary PCa, present in approximately 25% of the tumors, affects chromosome 8q, notably harboring the MYC oncogene.[3] Another frequent gain, present in around 10% of the cases, affects a region in the long arm of X chromosome, which contains the androgen

*Present address: Department of Experimental Gastroenterology, CIBERehd, Barcelona, Spain.

†Both authors have contributed equally to this study.

‡Dr. Ángel R. Ortiz died on May, 2008.

doi: 10.1111/j.1749-6632.2010.05780.x
Ann. N.Y. Acad. Sci. 1210 (2010) 17–24 © 2010 New York Academy of Sciences.

receptor gene and whose amplification has been suggested to be a tumoral mechanism to escape androgen withdrawal therapy and acquire androgen independence.[3,4] The most frequent deletion described in PCa so far is a loss in 8p21, found in more than 30% of the tumors.[3] This region carries the homeobox gene NKX3.1, whose loss of expression has been shown to correlate with tumor progression, being found in 20% of PIN lesions, 22% of T3 tumors, 34% of hormone refractory cases, and in almost 80% of metastases.[5] Another important tumor suppressor gene in PCa is the phosphatase and tensin homolog (PTEN) gene, located in 10q23, a region that is deleted in more than 10% of the tumors.[3] The loss of expression of PTEN correlates with high Gleason scores and advanced stages.[6] Other commonly deleted regions in prostate tumors include 13q in almost 30% of cases (with FOXO1A and the key cell cycle regulator RB1 as the most relevant genes) and 6q in 22% of the tumors (with FOXO3A, an apoptosis inducing gene).[3,7] However, many of the chromosomal gains and losses described in PCa are not consistently reported, or their frequencies vary widely between different studies. This apparent inconsistency is probably related to the inherent heterogeneity of prostate adenocarcinomas.

Unique to PCa are a group of microdeletions and rearrangements that cause the fusion of the untranslated 5' end of the androgen-regulated gene TMPRSS2 with several transcription factors of the ETS family, that result in the overexpression of the downstream transcription factor. These translocations have been found in approximately 60–70% of prostate tumors and 25% of PIN lesions.[8] About 50–80% of these rearrangements involve the ERG transcription factor and appear to associate with poor prognosis.[9] However, recent studies suggest that, although playing an important role in carcinogenesis, the TMPRSS2:ERG rearrangement is not sufficient for malignant transformation.[10]

The finding of genomic abnormalities in cancer gains functional significance when it is linked to differences in transcriptional activity. However, although there are numerous studies that have analyzed a variety of chromosomal abnormalities linked to PCa, few of them have explored the simultaneous analysis of structural (genomic) alterations and transcriptional or regulatory biochemical networks.[11–15] Table 1 shows chromosomal amplifications and deletions described in prostate tissue samples associated with differential transcriptional levels.[11,12] In an integrative genomic and transcriptomic analysis, Kim and colleagues showed that chromosomal alterations are only coupled to differences in gene expression in approximately 20% of the genes, both in tumoral and PIN lesions of the prostate.[11] This is an important consideration, since structural abnormalities are more likely to play important roles in carcinogenesis if they are reflected in altered transcriptional levels. The usual approach applied to associate structural and functional abnormalities in cancer has been to first generate genomic structural information from CGH or SNP array data, followed by, or together with, expression analysis to correlate the structural abnormalities with altered expression levels.[14–16] Nevertheless, these studies have shown low levels of concordance between genomic and transcriptomic data in PCa. It is possible that a reverse genetic approach could be a more efficient approach to find functionally significant chromosomal abnormalities. Similar strategies have been applied by others to study other neoplasias.[17–22]

Identification of a recurrent gain in PCa by the coordinate overexpression of genes located on chromosome 17q25.3

In a previous study,[23] we performed a transcriptomic analysis of prostate samples with the aim of finding gene expression changes in the tumoral glands that correlated with chromosomal abnormalities in the tumors. When performing transcriptional analysis with prostate samples, the high degree of tissue heterogeneity is a very important aspect to be taken into account, since it can lead to confounding results, highlighting genes whose differential expression is only the consequence of the different representation of cell compartments between benign and tumoral samples. Some studies have addressed this issue by applying *in silico* corrections to compensate for variable epithelial representations in different samples or by resorting to laser microdissection.[24,25] As an attempt to partially correct the biased results caused by prostate tissue heterogeneity, in addition to the normal and tumoral prostate samples under study, we included pure prostatic stromal samples and epithelial cell lines as representatives of these two compartments in order to be able to infer the specific expression pattern of epithelial and stromal cells. We analyzed

Table 1. Chromosomal alterations correlated with changes in transcript levels in human prostate tissue. Table shows amplified and deleted loci and selected genes in these regions that are over- or underexpressed, respectively.[11,12]

Locus	Correlated expression
Amplifications	Genes
1q21-q23	ARNT, FLG, GOLPH3L, LASS2, ADAM15, CRTC2, DPM3
1q32	MFSD4,NUCKS1
2q14	BUB1
3p25	ANKRD28
3q13	B4GALT4
3q26	GOLIM4,LRRC31,PDCD10,SERPINI1
5p15-p13	SKP2, SUB1
7p22	FOXK1, MMD2
7p14	SFRP4
7q32-q34	ATP6V1F, FLNC, MEST, SND1, BRAF,CALD1, TRIM24
8p11	AGPAT6,GINS4,GOLGA7
8q13	LACTB2,NCOA2,SLCO5A1,TRAM1, XKR9
8q22-q23	COX6C
9p13.3	UBAP1,UBAP2,UBE2R2,WDR40A
9q21-q34	C9orf5, DAPK1, NPDC1, SH3GLB2, TSC1, TTF1
11q13	CCND1, FGF4, DKFZp686L01105
13q32	ABCC4, ZIC2
16p12	CLN3, PALB2, PLK1
20q11	ID1, NCOA6
20q13	TSHZ2,ZNF217, CABLES2
Xq24-q26	ELF4, SLC25A5
Deletions	
1q21	ARNT, S100A2, SEC22B
1q25	HPC1, RNASEL, SOAT1
2q14-q23	BUB1, MGAT5, NMI
2q31	ITGA4, FLJ45259, SP3
3p13	RYBP,SHQ1, EIF4E3,FOXP1,PPP4R2
5p15	SRD5A1
5q11q12	ELOVL7, IL6ST, IQGAP2, MAP3K1, MSH3, PIK3R1,
5q21-q23	TNFAIP8, APC, CCNH, FER, GLRX
6p12-p11	BPAG1, ELOVL5, VEGFA, GSTA
6q12-q22	ATG5, CD164, COX7A2, EPHA7, FOXO3, HDAC2, SESN1
6q25-q27	IGF2R, SLC22A3, SOD2, TAB2, WTAP
7p15-p14	AQP1, HOXA13

Continued

Table 1. *Continued*

Locus	Correlated expression
8p21-p11	EGR3, EPB49, PPP3CC, BNIP3L, BRF2, CLU, NEFL, PPP2R2A
10q23-q24	PTEN, ACTA2, BMPR1A, MINPP1
12p13-p12	CD4, CDKN1B, DUSP16, ETV6, ING4, PRB2, PTPN6
13q12-q14	XPO4,LATS2,SAP18, C13orf18,LCP1,LRCH1,ZC3H13, P2RY5
14q13	C14orf24, FOXA1, SSTR1
15q13	GREM1, MEIS2
15q15	PDIA3, SORD, THBS1
16q23-q24	CDH13, FOXF1, MAF, WFDC1
17p13	ALOX15B, SAT2, TP53
17q21	GRN, HDAC5, LSM12, TMEM101, TMUB2, UBTF
18q11	LAMA3, CDH2, TAF4B
18q21	BCL2, NEDD4L, RAB27B, SMAD2
21q22	PSMG1, ERG,[a] FAM3B, HMGN1, ITGB2, PLAC4, SH3BGR
22q12-q13	CCDC117, FBLN1, HSCB, KDELR3, ST13

[a]Deletion in 21q22.2 results in the gene fusion *TM-PRSS2:ERG*.

microarray data by FADA, a method based on factor analysis that permits the identification of those genes that most significantly contribute to a given phenotype and to group the samples according to their degree of biological relatedness, while, importantly, allowing for the participation of one gene in more than one cluster, which better reflects actual biological networks.[26]

When applying FADA to the hybridization data, samples were clustered into their corresponding four biological groups of origin, namely, benign, tumoral, and stromal prostate tissue, and cell lines.[23] Our transcriptomic analysis by FADA also allowed the identification of the 318 genes showing the most significant differential expression between normal and tumoral tissues. One-hundred thirty four were overexpressed and 184 underexpressed in tumoral versus normal prostate tissues.[23]

Probably one of the most interesting features of expression profiling for thousands of genes is that they provide a panoramic view of the transcriptional status of a given sample. Taking advantage of this, we used FADA-selected genes to search for the possible colocalization of differentially expressed genes in adjacent positions in the genome, which can uncover higher levels of regulation that determine the selective coexpression of genes in tumoral samples. To determine putative nonrandom colocalizations of coexpressed genes, we determined the precise genomic localizations of all the genes present on the array (ENSEMBL-NCBI 36 assembly of the consensus human genome sequence). We then identified groups of four or more FADA-selected genes that were all either over- or underexpressed in tumoral samples and simultaneously colocalized in the genome within a distance of 4 Mb or fewer. From our analysis, the chromosomal region in which genes were coordinately overexpressed or underexpressed in tumors and showed the most significant colocalization was 17q25.3 ($P = 6.85 \times 10^{-4}$, Fig. 1A).[23] This region includes five genes selected by FADA as very significantly differentially expressed between normal and tumoral prostate samples, four of which colocalize on 17q25.3 within a segment of less than 0.4 Mb.

We reanalyzed the expression profiles of the genes in the 17q25.3 region present in the microarrays used in this study and found that their expression was epithelial-specific, since they were not expressed in stromal samples, and that most of the genes in this region were indeed overexpressed in a significant proportion of tumors compared to both normal and stromal tissues, even if they had not been selected in our original FADA analysis because of their lower discriminant power when taken individually (Fig. 1B).[23] Although comparative genomic hybridization studies by others had revealed gains in distal segments of 17q in some tumors, including PCa,[27,28] they had not been associated with the precise region in 17q25.3 described in our study or they had not been studied in specific detail. Our analysis suggests that this coordinated overexpression may be caused by a segmental chromosomal gain involving a region as small as 0.4 Mb in size, which may fall below the resolution of genome-wide BAC array-based CGH analysis.[29]

The causes for the relatively coordinated overexpression of so many genes that are so closely clustered in a small chromosomal region could be either genomic amplifications or gains of this region or, alternatively, the transcriptional coregulation by

factors acting in *trans*, or by a locus control region effect. In order to address this issue, we performed fluorescent *in situ* hybridization (FISH) on paraffin-embedded samples from the same 20 tumoral cases analyzed for their transcriptional profiles, hybridizing them with a BAC probe corresponding to the segment of interest on 17q25.3 (RP11–165M24) and a chromosome 17 centromeric probe. The results showed that there is indeed a gain in 17q25.3 in 65% (13/20) of the tumors analyzed, which harbored an average gain of three to four copies of this region (Fig. 2A, Ref. 23, and Table 2). The percentage of cells with a gain in 17q25.3 varied from 14% to 80%, with a mean of 47.4% nuclei containing the abnormality. The gain was found to be multifocal and present in some but not all the foci of a given tumor, which reflects the intrinsic heterogeneity of prostate tumors. Since we could only analyze some areas of these samples, this heterogeneity suggests that the observed prevalence of this segmental copy number gain is most likely an underestimate.

Interestingly, tumor-associated PIN lesions, precursors of PCa, also presented a gain in 17q25.3, which suggests that this chromosomal alteration represents an early event in prostate carcinogenesis (Fig. 2B,[23] Table 2). Furthermore, we also found the same gain in 65% (5/8) of the metastatic lesions analyzed, with a mean of 69.4% of nuclei containing the alteration (ranging from 47.5% to 98.5%). This observation involves this chromosomal alteration in all steps of progression of PCa (Fig. 2C,[23] Table 2): premalignant, malignant and metastatic.

Most of the genes in this region have been described to be involved in PCa or in other tumors. P4HB, for example, codes for a subunit of prolyl 4-hydroxylase and has been recently related to the stabilization of Argonaute-2, an important component of the RNA-induced silencing complex;[30] ARHGDIA codes for an inhibitor of GDP dissociation from the ras-like cytoskeleton regulator Rho;[31] ANAPC11 codes for an essential subunit of the anaphase-promoting complex;[32] SIRT7 codes for a homologue of the NAD$^+$-dependent histone deacetylase SIRT1 that regulates RNA polymerase III;[33] MAFG, whose product is a basic region leuzine-zipper transcription factor that heterodimerizes with NRF-2 to regulate the transcriptional response to oxidative stress, and also with Fos and JunB;[34,35] and ASPSCR1 (also known as ASPL), a gene frequently translocated in alveolar soft part

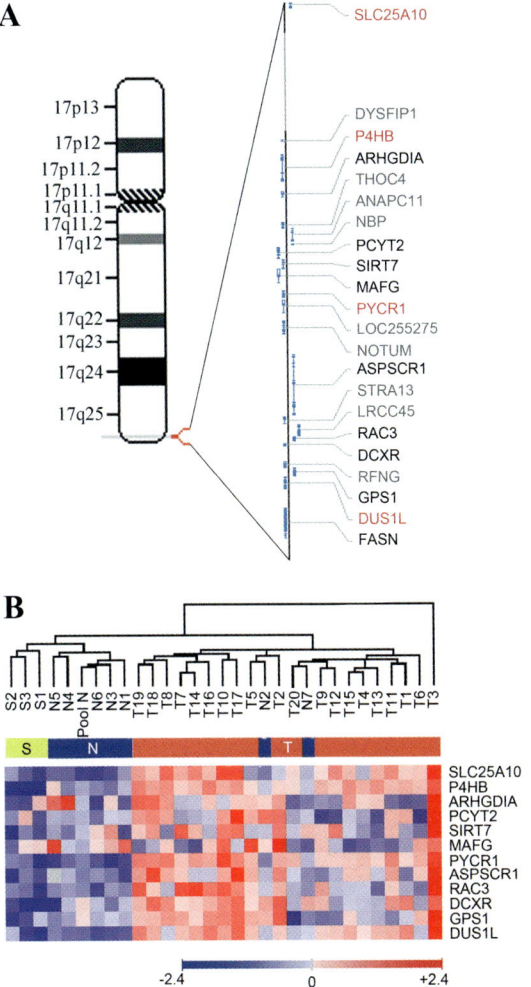

was found after analysis of the coordinated overexpression in tumors of the genes contained in this region, coupled to the functional involvement of many of these genes in the neoplastic process, reinforces the biological significance of this alteration in PCa.

The functional consequences of genomic abnormalities in cancer are mediated through altered functions of the encoded proteins and/or abnormal

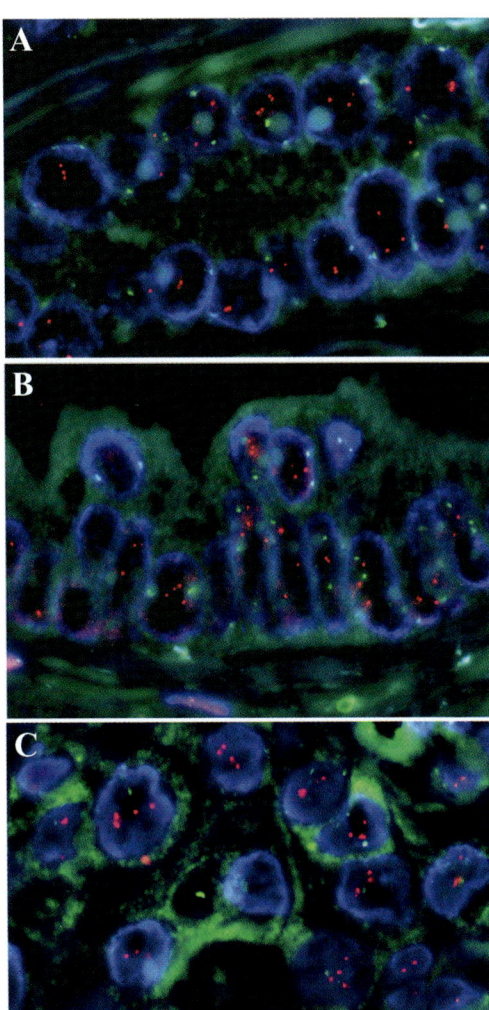

Figure 1. Prediction of a recurrent chromosomal gain in 17q25.3 in prostate tumors by transcript coregulation analysis. (A) Ideogram of chromosome 17 detailing the genes located on 17q25.3 with a corregulated overexpression in prostate cancer, as determined by our microarray analysis (red: genes selected by FADA as overexpressed in tumor samples; black: genes not selected by FADA but present in the Human Genome Focus microarrays; gray: genes not present in Human Genome Focus microarrays). (B) Heat map showing the relative expression levels of the genes on 17q25.3 shown in (A). The order of the genes is from centromeric (top panel) to telomeric (bottom panel). (Reported in Bermudo *et al.*[23]).

Figure 2. Experimental demonstration of a gain in 17q25.3 by fluorescent *in situ* hybridization in premalignant, malignant, and metastatic prostate samples. Images illustrating copy number gains in 17q25.3: selected representative regions of prostate carcinoma (A) and PIN (B) areas from the same sample, and a lymph node metastasis (C). Paraffin-embedded prostate samples were hybridized with the centromeric CEP17 probe (green) and the 17q25.3-specific BAC clone RP11–165M24 (red). (Reported in Bermudo *et al.*[23]).

sarcomas and papillary renal cell carcinomas to the chromosome X gene TFE3, causing the increased expression of this transcriptional regulator.[35] Also located in this region, immediately telomeric to DUS1L, is the fatty acid synthase gene (FASN), a well known marker of malignancy and progression in PC.[36] The fact that the recurrent gain in 17q25.3

Table 2. Results from the fluorescent *in situ* hybridization studies. Table shows the chromosomal status of the region 17q25.3 in the samples analyzed.

Case	Nuclei with a gain in 17q25.3 (%)	Number of copies of 17q25.3 (%)				
		2	3	4	>4	Polysomy
1	0	100	0	0	0	0
2	75	25	44	19.5	11.5	0
3	49	51	49	0	0	0
4	42.5	57.5	31.5	11	0	0
5	91	9	41.5	25	0	24.5
6	2	98	2	0	0	0
7	51.5	48.5	32	14	0	5.5
8	28	72.5	18.5	7.5	0	1.5
9	0.5	99.5	0.5	0	0	0
10	78	22	50	26.5	1.5	0
11	46	54	27.5	17.5	1	0
12	18	82	10	6.5	1.5	0
13	77	23	27.5	25.5	0	24
14	41.5	58.5	28.5	12.5	0.5	0
15	72	28	40	6.5	0	25.5
16	0	100	0	0	0	0
17	14	86	10	4	0	0
18	1	99	1	0	0	0
19	0	100	0	0	0	0
20	0	100	0	0	0	0

expression levels of the genes or noncoding RNAs located in regions of copy number alterations (CNAs). Thus, studying whether altered expression is due to CNAs by first analyzing coregulated transcription makes sense in that one focuses from the outset on those alterations most likely to be of functional relevance. We have shown that it is feasible to infer recurrent genomic alterations in cancer from transcriptomic data. Furthermore, the gain in 17q25.3 that our study has uncovered is one of the most highly prevalent chromosomal alterations thus far reported in PCa. These preliminary results warrant future studies with the inclusion of more cases, in order to establish the prevalence of this chromosomal alteration in PCa and to determine if its detection can have diagnostic or predictive value in this neoplasia.

Acknowledgments

This study was supported by grants from the Ministerio de Ciencia e Innovación (PI080274, SAF2008–04136), Ministerio de Educación y Ciencia (SAF2005–05109), Ministerio de Sanidad (PI020231), Red Temática de Cáncer of the Instituto Carlos III (ISCIII-RETIC RD06/0020), Xarxa de Bancs de Tumors de Catalunya-Pla Director d'Oncologia (XBTC-PDO), Fundació Marató TV3 and Fundación Ramón Areces.

Part of the results shown in this manuscript have been previously published in Bermudo *et al.* 2008. Coregulation analysis of closely linked genes identifies a highly recurrent gain on chromosome 17q25.3 in PCa. *BMC Cancer*, **8:** 315–326.

Author contributions

RB, TMT, and PLF have participated in the design, execution, analysis and writing of all the sections in this report. DA and ARO have participated in biocomputational analyses. DB and RV have participated in sample procurement. AC has contributed to FISH analysis.

Conflicts of interest

The authors declare no conflicts of interest.

References

1. Ferlay, J., F. Bray, P. Pisani & D.M. Parkin. 2004. *GLOBOCAN 2002. Cancer Incidence, Mortality and Prevalence Worldwide. IARC CancerBase No. 5 (version 2.0).* IARC Press. Lyon.

2. Hughes, S., M. Yoshimoto, B. Beheshti, *et al.* 2006. The use of whole genome amplification to study chromosomal changes in prostate cancer: insights into genome-wide signature of preneoplasia associated with cancer progression. *BMC Genomics* **7:** 65–74.

3. Sun, J., W. Liu, T.S. Adams, *et al.* 2007. DNA copy number alterations in prostate cancers: a combined analysis of published CGH studies. *Prostate* **67:** 692–700.

4. Visakorpi, T., E. Hyytinen, P. Koivisto, *et al.* 1995. In vivo amplification of the androgen receptor gene and progression of human prostate cancer. *Nat. Genet.* **9:** 401–406.

5. Bowen, C., L. Bubendorf, H.J. Voeller, *et al.* 2000. Loss of NKX3.1 expression in human prostate cancers correlates with tumor progression. *Cancer Res.* **60:** 6111–6115.

6. McMenamin, M.E., P. Soung, S. Perera, *et al.* 1999. Loss of PTEN expression in paraffin-embedded primary prostate cancer correlates with high Gleason score and advanced stage. *Cancer Res.* **59:** 4291–4296.

7. Trotman, L.C., A. Alimonti, P.P. Scaglioni, *et al.* 2006. Identification of a tumour suppressor network opposing nuclear Akt function. *Nature* **441:** 523–527.

8. Tomlins, S.A., D.R. Rhodes, S. Perner, *et al.* 2005. Recurrent fusion of TMPRSS2 and ETS transcription factor genes in prostate cancer. *Science* **310:** 644–648.

9. Demichelis, F., K. Fall, S. Perner, *et al.* 2007. TMPRSS2: ERG gene fusion associated with lethal prostate cancer in a watchful waiting cohort. *Oncogene* **26:** 4596–4599.

10. Tomlins, S.A., B. Laxman, S. Varambally, *et al.* 2008. Role of the TMPRSS2-ERG gene fusion in prostate cancer. *Neoplasia* **10:** 177–188.

11. Kim, J.H., S.M. Dhanasekaran, R. Mehra, *et al.* 2007. Integrative analysis of genomic aberrations associated with prostate cancer progression. *Cancer Res.* **67:** 8229–8239.

12. Taylor, B.S., N. Schultz, H. Hieronymus, *et al.* Integrative genomic profiling of human prostate cancer. *Cancer Cell.* **18:** 11–22.

13. Chaudhary, J. & M. Schmidt. 2006. The impact of genomic alterations on the transcriptome: a prostate cancer cell line case study. *Chromosome Res.* **14:** 567–586.

14. Wolf, M., S. Mousses, S. Hautaniemi, *et al.* 2004. High-resolution analysis of gene copy number alterations in human prostate cancer using CGH on cDNA microarrays: impact of copy number on gene expression. *Neoplasia* **6:** 240–247.

15. Zhao, H., Y. Kim, P. Wang, *et al.* 2005. Genome-wide characterization of gene expression variations and DNA copy number changes in prostate cancer cell lines. *Prostate* **63:** 187–197.

16. Saramaki, O.R., K.P. Porkka, R.L. Vessella & T. Visakorpi. 2006. Genetic aberrations in prostate cancer by microarray analysis. *Int. J. Cancer* **119:** 1322–1329.

17. Dressman, M.A., A. Baras, R. Malinowski, *et al.* 2003. Gene expression profiling detects gene amplification and differentiates tumor types in breast cancer. *Cancer Res.* **63:** 2194–2199.

18. Grade, M., P. Hormann, S. Becker, *et al.* 2007. Gene expression profiling reveals a massive, aneuploidy-dependent transcriptional deregulation and distinct differences between lymph node-negative and lymph node-positive colon carcinomas. *Cancer Res.* **67:** 41–56.

19. Fritz, B., F. Schubert, G. Wrobel, *et al.* 2002. Microarray-based copy number and expression profiling in dedifferentiated and pleomorphic liposarcoma. *Cancer Res.* **62:** 2993–2998.

20. Pollack, J.R., T. Sorlie, C.M. Perou, *et al.* 2002. Microarray analysis reveals a major direct role of DNA copy number alteration in the transcriptional program of human breast tumors. *Proc. Natl. Acad. Sci. USA* **99:** 12963–12968.

21. Tonon, G., K.K. Wong, G. Maulik, *et al.* 2005. High-resolution genomic profiles of human lung cancer. *Proc. Natl. Acad. Sci. USA* **102:** 9625–9630.

22. Aguirre, A.J., C. Brennan, G. Bailey, *et al.* 2004. High-resolution characterization of the pancreatic adenocarcinoma genome. *Proc. Natl. Acad. Sci. USA* **101:** 9067–9072.

23. Bermudo, R., D. Abia, B. Ferrer, *et al.* 2008. Co-regulation analysis of closely linked genes identifies a highly recurrent gain on chromosome 17q25.3 in prostate cancer. *BMC Cancer* **8:** 315–326.

24. Ernst, T., M. Hergenhahn, M. Kenzelmann, *et al.* 2002. Decrease and gain of gene expression are equally discriminatory markers for prostate carcinoma: a gene expression analysis on total and microdissected prostate tissue. *Am. J. Pathol.* **160:** 2169–2180.

25. Stuart, R.O., W. Wachsman, C.C. Berry, *et al.* 2004. In silico dissection of cell-type-associated patterns of gene expression in prostate cancer. *Proc. Natl. Acad. Sci. USA* **101:** 615–620.

26. Lozano, J.J., M. Soler, R. Bermudo, *et al.* 2005. Dual activation of pathways regulated by steroid receptors and peptide growth factors in primary prostate cancer revealed by Factor Analysis of microarray data. *BMC Genomics* **6:** 109–126.

27. Shah, U.S., R. Dhir, S.M. Gollin, *et al.* 2006. Fatty acid synthase gene overexpression and copy number gain in prostate adenocarcinoma. *Hum. Pathol.* **37:** 401–409.

28. Storlazzi, C.T., H.R. Brekke, N. Mandahl, *et al.* 2006. Identification of a novel amplicon at distal 17q containing the BIRC5/SURVIVIN gene in malignant peripheral nerve sheath tumours. *J. Pathol.* **209:** 492–500.

29. Greshock, J., T.L. Naylor, A. Margolin, *et al.* 2004. 1-Mb resolution array-based comparative genomic hybridization using a BAC clone set optimized for cancer gene analysis. *Genome Res.* **14:** 179–187.

30. Qi, H.H., P.P. Öngusaha, J. Myllyharju, *et al.* 2008. Prolyl 4-hydroxylation regulates Argonaute 2 stability. *Nature* **455:** 421–424.

31. Malliri, A. & J.G. Collard. 2003. Role of Rho-family proteins in cell adhesion and cancer. *Curr. Opin. Cell Biol.* **15:** 583–589.

32. Peters, J.M. 2006. The anaphase promoting complex/ cyclosome: a machine designed to destroy. *Nat. Rev. Mol. Cell Biol.* **7:** 644–656.

33. Lapointe, J., C. Li, J.P. Higgins, *et al.* 2004. Gene expression profiling identifies clinically relevant subtypes of prostate cancer. *Proc. Natl. Acad. Sci. USA* **101:** 811–816.

34. Katsuoka, F., H. Motohashi, J.D. Engel & M. Yamamoto. 2005. Nrf2 transcriptionally activates the mafG gene through an antioxidant response element. *J. Biol. Chem.* **280:** 4483–4490.

35. Ladanyi, M., M.Y. Lui, C.R. Antonescu, *et al.* 2001. The der(17)t(X;17)(p11;q25) of human alveolar soft part sarcoma fuses the TFE3 transcription factor gene to ASPL, a novel gene at 17q25. *Oncogene* **20:** 48–57.

36. Kuhajda, F.P. 2006. Fatty acid synthase and cancer: new application of an old pathway. *Cancer Res.* **66:** 5977–5980.

Ann. N.Y. Acad. Sci. ISSN 0077-8923

ANNALS OF THE NEW YORK ACADEMY OF SCIENCES
Issue: *Toward Personalized Medicine for Cancer*

MicroRNAs in cancer: personalizing diagnosis and therapy

S. Patrick Nana-Sinkam,[1,3] Muller Fabbri,[2,3] and Carlo M. Croce[2,3]

[1]Division of Pulmonary, Allergy, Critical Care and Sleep Medicine, The Ohio State University, Columbus, Ohio. [2]Department of Molecular Virology, Immunology, and Medical Genetics, The Ohio State University, Columbus, Ohio. [3]James Comprehensive Cancer Center, The Ohio State University, Columbus, Ohio

Address for correspondence: Carlo M. Croce, M.D., Department of Molecular Virology, Immunology and Medical Genetics, The Ohio State University, 410 West 10th Avenue, Columbus, OH 43210. Carlo.Croce@osumc.edu

MicroRNAs (miRNAs) are 19–24nt noncoding RNAs that have been implicated in the pathogenesis of both solid and hematological malignancies. Frequently located in fragile chromosomal regions, miRNAs are essential to key biological functions, such as cellular differentiation, apoptosis, and growth. miRNAs may serve as either tumor suppressors or oncogenes. As a result, they have the potential to serve as both biomarkers and therapeutic agents in cancer. Based on our presentation at the recent Towards Personalized Cancer Medicine conference held in Barcelona, Spain, May 19–21, 2010, we provide an overview of the current knowledge of miRNA deregulation in solid and hematological malignancies and their application as biomarkers of disease.

Keywords: microRNA; cancer; biomarkers; genome

Introduction

It is estimated that 12.7 million new cancer cases and 7.6 million deaths occurred in 2008.[1] Thus, cancer remains a global epidemic with significant socio-economic impact.[1] There are multiple components to fighting the battle against cancer, including but not limited to, elucidating the molecular mechanisms of cancer cell behavior, novel targeted therapeutic development, biomarker discovery, early detection, and risk modification. It is increasingly clear that many cancers are heterogenous in terms of their molecular signatures and clinical manifestations. Linking these genotypic differences to clinical phenotype is both complex and necessary for the development of novel therapies.

First identified in 1993, MicroRNAs (miRNAs or miRs) are noncoding RNAs essential to basic biological functions such as growth, invasion, angiogenesis, proliferation, and differentiation.[2,3] MiRNAs are often located in fragile chromosome regions that are susceptible to deletions, amplifications and translocations.[4] By targeting the 3′ and 5′ untranslated regions (UTR), miRNAs may regulate tens to hundreds of genes.[4] It is estimated that miRNAs are responsible for the regulation of over one third of

the genome and that miRNAs may function as either oncogenes or tumor suppressors.[4] Dysregulation of miRNA expression has been described in several solid and hematological malignancies(Figure 1). This observation combined with both *in vivo* and *in vitro* allied studies demonstrating functionality supports their importance to the pathogenesis of cancer. MiRNAs are emerging as diagnostic and prognostic biomarkers as well as potential therapeutic targets in the battle against cancer.

MiRNAs in hematological malignancies

In hematologic malignancies, miRNA expression levels can be successfully used as diagnostic and prognostic biomarkers. Table 1 summarizes the most frequently deregulated miRNAs in hematologic malignancies with the diagnostic/prognostic implications of the observed deregulation. In chronic lymphocytic leukemia (CLL), low levels of *miR-15a/16–1* are associated with the indolent form of the disease (characterized by low levels of Zap-70 and IgV$_H$ mutated status),[5] whereas low levels of *miR-29*b and *miR-181b* correlate with aggressive CLL, overexpressing their direct target TCL1.[6] In Philadelphia positive chronic myelocytic

doi: 10.1111/j.1749-6632.2010.05822.x

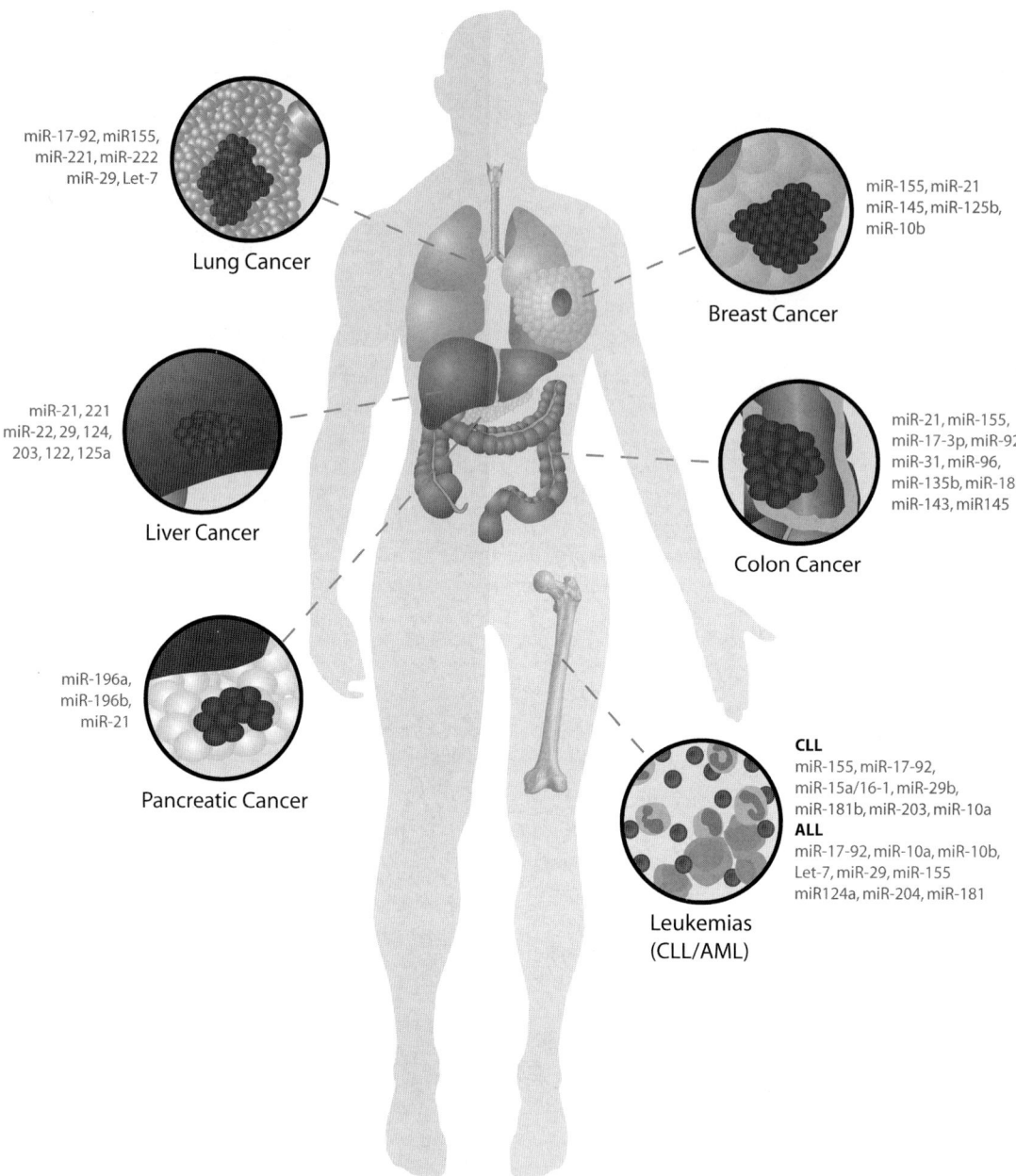

Figure 1. Deregulated miRNA in cancer: red represents increased miRNA, and blues are decreased miRNA.

leukemia (CML), overexpression of the *miR-17–92* cluster occurs as an early event,[7] whereas low levels of *miR-203*[8] and *miR-10a*[9] complete the so-far decoded diagnostic signature of CML. Upregulation of the *miR-17–92* cluster was documented also in acute lymphoblastic leukemia (ALL),[10] a disease in which *miR-124a* is frequently downregulated because of promoter hypermethylation.[11]

In acute myeloblastic leukemia (AML) a signature composed of high expression of *miR-10a*, *-10b*, several *let-7*, and *miR-29* family members and low expression of *miR-204* is a hallmark of AML with mutated NPM1 (nuclephosmin-1), whereas high levels of *miR-155* are more frequently found in AML with FLT3-ITD+ status.[12] From the prognostic point of view, AML patients with low levels of *miR-181*

Table 1. Most frequently deregulated miRNAs in hematologic malignancies

Disease	Downregulation	Upregulation
CLL	*miR-15a/16–1* cluster (indolent) *miR-29b, miR-181b* (aggressive)	*miR-155* (aggressive)
CML	*miR-203* *miR-10a*	*miR-17–92* cluster
ALL	*miR-124a*	*miR-17–92* cluster
AML	*miR-204* (NPM1 mut) *miR-181* (FLT3-ITD+ and/or NPM1 mut)	*miR-10a* *miR-10b* let-7 family *miR-29* family *miR-155* (FLT3-ITD+) *miR-191* (poor prognosis) *miR-199a* (poor prognosis)
BL		*miR-155*
DLBCL		*miR-155* (ABC-DLBCL)
HL	*miR-135a* (poor prognosis)	*miR-155*

CLL, chronic lymphocytic leukemia; CML, chronic myelocytic leukemia; ALL, acute lymphoblastic leukemia; AML, acute myeloblastic leukemia; BL, Burkitt lymphoma; DLBCL, diffuse large B cell lymphoma; HL, Hodgkin lymphoma; NPM1 mut, mutated nucleophosmin-1; FLT3-ITD+, FMS-like tyrosine kinase 3/internal ndem duplication; ABC-DLBCL, activated B cell phenotype diffuse large B cell lymphoma.

family experience a more aggressive phenotype of the disease (FLT-ITD+, or unmutated NPM1, or both),[13] and high expression of *miR-191* and *-199a* correlates with reduced overall and disease-free survival in AML.[14] Interestingly, a panel of four miRNAs was able to distinguish between ALL and AML with high accuracy (about 98%): upregulation of *miR-128a* and *-128b* suggest ALL, whereas upregulation of *miR-223* and *let-7b* are suggestive of a diagnosis of AML.[15] With the same high level of accuracy, four miRNAs (namely *miR-330, -17–5p, -106a,* and *-210*) can differentiate between reactive lymph nodes, follicular lymphomas and diffuse large B cell lymphomas (DLBCL).[16] Moreover, high levels of *miR-155* are associated with the activated B cell phenotype of DLBCL (ABC-DLBCL),[17,18] which is the variant of DLBCL with the shorter overall survival,[19] indicating that *miR-155* has a prognostic significance in DLBCL. Also in Hodgkin lymphoma (HL), specific miRNA diagnostic signatures have been identified,[20,21] and low expression of *miR-135a* has been associated with higher relapse risk and shorter disease-free survival.[22]

Overall, several miRNAs are deregulated in hematologic malignancies (for a review, see Refs. 23–25). For some of these most frequently deregulated miRNAs, genetically engineered animal models are available. These models may provide information on the causal relationships of specific genetic alterations found in these malignancies, and may serve as an invaluable tool to test novel therapies. In hematologic malignancies three groups of miRNAs are frequently deregulated, which has led to the development of animal models that have in turn clarified their role in these tumors: the *miR-15a/16–1* cluster, the *miR-17–92* cluster and *miR-155* mouse models.

CLL is the most common form of leukemia of the adult in the Western world.[26] This disease is characterized by recurrent chromosomal abnormalities, the most frequent of which is the deletion of the 13q14.3 region.[27] Interestingly, the deletion affects the expression of a cluster of miRNAs (the *miR-15a/16–1* cluster),[28] which directly target BCL2,[29,30] an anti-apoptotic gene overexpressed in the majority of indolent CLLs. These findings support a role for the *miR-15a/16–1* cluster in CLL pathogenesis. Given the fact that validated CLL cell lines are currently not available, mouse models are important to the study of human CLL.[31] The New Zealand Black (NZB) strain is characterized by naturally occurring late-onset CLL and a clonal expansion of a subpopulation of B cells (called B-1) that resemble human CLL.[32] Intriguingly, DNA sequencing from multiple NZB tissues detected a C→T point mutation in the 3'-flanking region of the precursor of *miR-16-1*,[33] very similar to the point mutation described in *miR-16–1* 3'-flanking sequence of two CLL patients (one of whom with a history of familial CLL and breast cancer).[5] In the NZB model, the point mutation was responsible for reduced expression of *miR-16*, and restoration of this miRNA in a NZB malignant CLL cell line resulted in a G1 arrest, and decreased number of cells in S phase.[33] Recently, Klein and colleagues[34] have developed a mouse model that carries conditional alleles, mimicking the deletion of the minimal deleted region (MDR), previously described in human CLL,[35,36] and comprising either the entire DLEU2 gene (which provides the primary transcript for the *miR-15a/16–1* cluster), or selectively the *miR-15a/16–1* cluster, without affecting the expression of DLEU2. They showed that both deletions lead to lymphoproliferative disorders with an indolent course resembling that of human CLL with 13q deletion, but MDR[−/−] mice displayed a more aggressive phenotype.[30] These findings suggest that other genes (in addition to the *miR-15a/16–1* cluster itself) contribute to the tumor suppressor role of the MDR locus, and indicate that the noncoding RNA produced by DLEU2 itself might have regulatory functions. In this same study, the authors also showed that the *miR-15a/16–1* cluster exerts its antitumoral effect on human and mouse B cells by downregulating several genes involved in the G0/G1-S phase transition, whereas no impairment in cell proliferation was observed upon restoration of DLEU2 expression.[30] These data are consistent with the results of Salerno and colleagues, who showed that when *miR-15a/16–1* are re-expressed in the B1 cells of NZB mice, a reduction of cyclin D1 occurs, leading to a block of the G0/G1-S transition.[37]

The *miR-17–92* cluster maps at chromosome 13q31–32, in a region that is frequently amplified in malignant B cell lymphomas[38] and is overexpressed in more than 60% of B cell lymphoma patients.[39] The oncogenic potential of this cluster is corroborated by experimental evidence that its retroviral expression in hematopoietic cells accelerates the onset of c-Myc-mediated lymphomagenesis in a TG mouse model involving bone marrow reconstitution.[38] Xiao and colleagues showed that *miR-17–92* TG mouse models develop a higher than expected rate of lymphoproliferative and autoimmune disorders, and undergo a premature death.[40] These oncogenic effects are at least in part explained by the direct targeting effect on the two tumor suppressor genes PTEN and BIM, which control B-lymphocyte apoptosis.[40] The work by Ventura and colleagues has demonstrated that the *miR-17–92* cluster function overlaps with that of its paralogous *miR-106b–25* cluster on chromosome 7. In fact, the *miR-17–92* and *miR-106b-25* double KO mouse model develops a more severe phenotype than the *miR-17–92* single KO model.[41] More recently, it has been demonstrated that the real culprit of the oncogenic transformation within the *miR-17–92* cluster is *miR-19*. In the Eu-Myc model of Burkitt lymphoma, *miR-19* is both necessary and sufficient for *miR-17–92* cluster to promote c-Myc induced B lymphomagenesis. In particular, *miR-19* acts by targeting PTEN and activates the PI3K-Akt-mTOR pathway leading to increased carcinogenesis.[42] These results were confirmed by Mu and colleagues, in a mouse model characterized by conditional loss of function of the m*iR-17–92* cluster.[43]

High levels of *miR-155* have been described in several human malignancies (both solid and hematologic).[44,45] Specifically, upregulation of *miR-155* occurs in CLL,[46] Burkitt lymphoma,[47] DLBCL 16,18 and HL 21.[48,49] To better understand the role of *miR-155* in leukemias/lymphomas, both transgenic (TG) and knockout (KO) mouse models have been generated. Costinean and colleagues developed the first B cell-specific *miR-155* TG mouse. At the age of approximately 9 months, these mice develop an ALL/high-grade lymphoma, preceded by a polyclonal pre-B cell proliferation.[50] A further characterization of these mice showed that the B cell precursors with the highest expression of *miR-155* were indeed at the origin of the leukemias, because this miRNA directly targets SHIP (Src homology 2 domain-containing inositol-5-phosphate), and C/EBPbeta (CCAAT enhancer-binding protein beta), two inhibitors of IL-6, leading to a block in pre-B cell differentiation.[51] In *miR-155* KO models, impairment of the antibody affinity maturation and of memory B cell generation in a T cell–dependent antibody response have been described.[52,53] Moreover, *miR-155* ablation resulted in reduced extra follicular and germinal center responses and impaired the memory response.[52,53]

In summary, the development of therapeutic tools targeting the overexpression of *miR-17–92* cluster and *miR-155*, and restoring normal levels of *miR-15a/16–1* in haematological malignancies might impact the molecular pathogenetic mechanisms of these diseases, therefore representing a promising novel approach to the treatment of human leukemias/lymphomas.

Colorectal cancer

The miRNA diagnostic signature for colorectal cancer (CRC) is characterized by high levels of *miR-31, -96, -135b,* and *-183,*[54] and low levels of *miR-143* and *-145,*[55] whereas higher expression of *miR-21* is more frequently associated with stage Dukes C, than stages A and B.[56] Interestingly, it has also been demonstrated that specific miRNA patterns of expression are able to identify the occurrence of microsatellite instability in CRC at the time of diagnosis.[57] High levels of *miR-155* have been described also in CRC tissues with respect to the normal counterpart,[44] and recently it has been demonstrated that high levels of *miR-155* increase microsatellite instability by direct targeting of key mismatch repair genes: MLH1, MSH2, and MSH6.[58] The recently increasing interest in the detection of circulating miRNAs has led to the use of miRNAs as diagnostic and prognostic biomarkers in CRC. A study by Chen and colleagues demonstrated that 69 miRNAs are differentially expressed in the serum of CRC patients with respect to non cancerous patients.[59] In particular, high levels of *miR-17–3p* and *miR-92* were consistently elevated in CRC and were significantly reduced in 10 patients after surgery, corroborating their valuable use as tumor circulating biomarkers.[60]

Pancreatic cancer

A signature of 25 deregulated miRNAs (21 upregulated and 4 downregulated) was able to differentiate between pancreatic adenocarcinoma, chronic pancreatitis and normal pancreas.[61] High expression of *miR-196a* and *-196b* was suggestive of a diagnosis of pancreatic ductal adenocarcinoma because this overexpression does not occur in normal or inflamed pancreatic tissue.[62] Interestingly, *miR-196a* was not detectable in normal acinar pancreatic cells, but only in ductal adenocarcinoma cells of the pancreas, and the expression level of this miRNA parallels pancreatic cancer ductal carcinoma progression.[63] Recently, it has been demonstrated that patients with high *miR-21* expression had a significantly shorter overall survival both in the metastatic and in the adjuvant setting.[64] Moreover, high expression of *miR-21* conferred chemoresistance to gemcitabine, which is currently one of the most effective drugs in the treatment of pancreatic ductal adenocarcinoma.[64,65] Despite the fact that no conditional mouse model has been developed yet to specifically address the role of miRNAs in pancreatic cancer, there is clear evidence of their involvement in the pathogenesis of this disease, and further studies are warranted to investigate the effect of miRNA silencing/restoring treatments as effective weapons against this still very lethal tumor.

Lung cancer

Lung cancer is the number one cause of cancer related deaths among men and women.[66] It is estimated that in 2010, there will be 222,520 new cases of lung cancer and 157,300 deaths in the United States. Deregulation of miRNAs in lung cancer has been described in several studies. Global deregulation of miRNAs also coorelates with survival in lung cancer. Yanaihara and colleagues identified 43 differentially expressed miRNAs between lung tumors and adjacent uninvolved lung.[67] Both elevated *miR-155* and low *let7a-2* expression correlated with worse survival. In a separate independent study, investigators identified both high-risk miRNAs (*miR-137, -182*,* and *-372*) that increased the invasive capacity in cancer cells and protective miRNAs, such as *miR-221*, which decreased invasion that correlated with overall disease-free survival in a cohort of 122 patients with NSCLC.[68]

The *miR-29* family functionally targets DNA methyltransferases (DNMT) 3A and -3B, two key enzymes involved in DNA methylation, and is often increased in malignancies such as lung cancer.[69] High DNMT3A correlated with worse overall survival in lung cancer.[69] Gain of function of *miR-29* homologs in lung cancer cells restored DNA methylation patterns and the expression of tumor suppressors such as both FHIT and WWOX expression. In addition, *miR-29a*, b, and c reduced tumor development in a murine xenograft model.[69]

Garofalo and colleagues recently demonstrated that *miR-222* and *miR-222* are inversely correlated with expression of both tumor suppressors PTEN and TIMP3 in hepatocellular carcinoma and lung cancer.[70] *MiR-221* and *miR-222* are induced by the MET oncogene. *MiR-221* and *222* functionally target PTEN and TIMP3 to induce cancer cell migratory and invasive capacity.[70] Lastly, both *miR-221* and *miR-222* were upregulated in TNF-α related apoptosis-inducing ligand cell lines. Silencing of these miRNAs sensitized resistant cell lines to TRAIL agents.[70]

Let-7 is one miRNA that has been extensively studied in cancer.[71,72] *Let-7* targets the RAS 3′UTR and inhibits tumor growth.[72] Transgenic murine models of lung cancer demonstrated that *Let-7* overexpression inhibited tumor development and growth.[71]

Breast cancer

One of the earliest studies to examine global deregulation of miRNAs in breast cancer demonstrated in 76 breast cancers and 10 normal breast tissues that 29 miRNAs were aberrantly expressed. *MiR-155* (increased), *miR-21* (increased), *miR-145* (decreased), *miR-125b* (decreased), and *miR-10b* (decreased) were the most deregulated miRNAs.[73] In addition, the authors identified an association between select deregulated miRNA and pathological features such as estrogen and progesterone receptor positivity, lymph node metastases, and presence of vascular invasion. Because that initial observation, each of these miRNAs has been studied and validated as being of functional relevance in breast cancer. *MiR-145* is deregulated in several cancers. *MiR-145* reduced breast cancer cell proliferation and induced apoptosis.[74] These effects were partially mediated through TP53 pathway activation and targeting of the estrogen receptor α (ER-α) 74. *MiR-145* also targets genes critical to invasion and metastases including mucin-1.[75]

MiR-155 is frequently upregulated in several malignancies including breast cancer, thus suggesting its role as an oncogene. In addition, it may serve as a critical link between the inflammatory process and development of cancer.[76] Its correlation with tumor progression and survival makes it an attractive candidate for therapy. In breast cancer, investigators demonstrated *in vitro* that *miR-155* confers chemoresistance through targeting of the forkhead transcription factor FOXO3a.[77] Selective *miR-155* knockdown rendered the cells chemosensitive. A recent study identified the suppressor of cytokine signaling (socs1) as a target for *miR-155* and essential to the pro-proliferative effects of *miR-155*.[78]

miRNA networks in cancer

As the number of miRNAs in the human genome has approached 1,000, it has become increasingly clear that the miRNA regulation of a specific target gene, protein, cellular behavior, and ultimately development of disease is highly complex. Although the reductionist approach of investigating single miRNA single target gene relationships is of value, tumor initiation and progression is likely dependent on multiple miRNAs and genes. Therefore, the integration of both miRNA and target gene patterns of expression to then identify "network" deregulation is critical to our understanding of the role that miRNAs play both as biomarkers and therapeutic targets. We recently examined the patterns of miRNA expression in 4,419 human tissues.[79] Among 17 groups of human normal tissues and 1,107 total samples, we identified clusters of miRNAs that were linked by similar cellular functions. For example, *miR-1* and *miR-133a/b* were linked. They are involved in muscle differentiation and proliferation. *MiR-29* was linked to *miR-30* and *miR-15/16*. All miRNAs target prosurvival molecules. We then conducted a similar examination within 51 cancer types for a total of 3,312 samples (2,532 solid cancers and 780 leukemia samples).[79] A comparison between solid cancers and normal tissues confirmed upregulation of miRNAs (*miR-21, miR-25, miR-17*, and *miR-92a*) and downregulation (*miR-145* and *miR-205*) previously described in individual cancers. The most common pathways identified by KEGG analysis of deregulated miRNAs in cancers included the Wnt, phosphatidylinositol, focal adhesion, and VEGF pathways. When directly comparing miRNA networks of normal tissues to those of solid cancers, we identified differences in representation of miRNA hubs. For example, in cancers, *miR-30c* was highly linked whereas in normal tissues it was not. Applying this approach to specific cancers (e.g., lung cancer and acute myeloid leukemia), we were able to detect differences not only in distribution of miRNAs but also in the numbers of networks.[79] Normal lung was characterized by one interconnected network of miRNAs whereas adenocarcinoma of the lung had one large interconnected network and eight nonconnected networks.[79] An important finding was that several solid malignancies harbored similar nonconnected miRNAs (e.g., *miR-10a/b* and *miR-29a/b* in breast, colon, and lung cancer; *let-7c/a* in colon, lung, and prostate cancers). Leukemias also harbored distinct miRNA networks with AML having two networks with *miR-155* and *miR-181* being separate. In CLL, there was one large network with two separate networks. The smaller networks involved *miR-15a/16* and *miR-23*. This corroborates previous literature demonstrating *miR-15a/16* as an important component of pathogenesis of CLL.

Conclusion

The journey from the initial observations that regulatory RNAs are critical to larval development to the current application of this same class of noncoding RNAs as biomarkers and potential targets in human cancer has been both interesting and complex. The global deregulation of miRNAs across cancers including leukemias, colon cancer, pancreatic cancer, lung, and breast cancer to name a few clearly demonstrates fundamental importance to disease initiation and progression. Although individual miRNA/target relationships are critical to our understanding, a global view of aberrant miRNA networks between normal and cancer and between cancers is of equal importance. It is anticipated that such studies may be used to identify both tumor type specific miRNAs and links between miRNAs and molecular pathways that can then be exploited for therapeutic application.

Acknowledgment

The authors would like to thank Dr. Tim Eubank for his assistance in the preparation of the figure.

Conflicts of interest

The authors declare no conflicts of interest.

References

1. International Agency for Research on Cancer. GLOBOCAN 2008. http://globocan.iarc.fr/.
2. Lee, R.C., R.L. Feinbaum & V. Ambros. 1993. The *C. elegans* heterochronic gene lin-4 encodes small RNAs with antisense complementarity to lin-14. *Cell* **75:** 843–854.
3. Bartel, D.P. 2004. MicroRNAs: genomics, biogenesis, mechanism, and function. *Cell* **116:** 281–297.
4. Croce, C.M. 2009. Causes and consequences of microRNA dysregulation in cancer. *Nat. Rev. Genet.* **10:** 704–714.

5. Calin, G.A., M. Ferracin, A. Cimmino, *et al.* 2005. A MicroRNA signature associated with prognosis and progression in chronic lymphocytic leukemia. *N. Engl. J. Med.* **353:** 1793–1801.
6. Pekarsky, Y., U. Santanam, A. Cimmino, *et al.* 2006. Tcl1 expression in chronic lymphocytic leukemia is regulated by miR-29 and miR-181. *Cancer Res.* **66:** 11590–11593.
7. Venturini, L., K. Battmer, M. Castoldi, *et al.* 2007. Expression of the miR-17–92 polycistron in chronic myeloid leukemia (CML) CD34+ cells. *Blood* **109:** 4399–4405.
8. Bueno, M.J., I. Perez de Castro, M. Gomez de Cedron, *et al.* 2008. Genetic and epigenetic silencing of microRNA-203 enhances ABL1 and BCR-ABL1 oncogene expression. *Cancer Cell* **13:** 496–506.
9. Agirre, X., A. Jimenez-Velasco, E. San Jose-Eneriz, *et al.* 2008. Down-regulation of hsa-miR-10a in chronic myeloid leukemia CD34+ cells increases USF2-mediated cell growth. *Mol. Cancer Res.* **6:** 1830–1840.
10. Zanette, D.L., F. Rivadavia, G.A. Molfetta, *et al.* 2007. miRNA expression profiles in chronic lymphocytic and acute lymphocytic leukemia. *Braz. J. Med. Biol. Res.* **40:** 1435–1440.
11. Agirre, X., A. Vilas-Zornoza, A. Jimenez-Velasco, *et al.* 2009. Epigenetic silencing of the tumor suppressor microRNA Hsa-miR-124a regulates CDK6 expression and confers a poor prognosis in acute lymphoblastic leukemia. *Cancer Res.* **69:** 4443–4453.
12. Garzon, R., M. Garofalo, M.P. Martelli, *et al.* 2008. Distinctive microRNA signature of acute myeloid leukemia bearing cytoplasmic mutated nucleophosmin. *Proc. Natl. Acad. Sci. USA* **105:** 3945–3950.
13. Marcucci, G., M.D. Radmacher, K. Maharry, *et al.* 2008. MicroRNA expression in cytogenetically normal acute myeloid leukemia. *N. Engl. J. Med.* **358:** 1919–1928.
14. Garzon, R., S. Volinia, C.G. Liu, *et al.* 2008. MicroRNA signatures associated with cytogenetics and prognosis in acute myeloid leukemia. *Blood* **111:** 3183–3189.
15. Mi, S., J. Lu, M. Sun, *et al.* 2007. MicroRNA expression signatures accurately discriminate acute lymphoblastic leukemia from acute myeloid leukemia. *Proc. Natl. Acad. Sci. USA* **104:** 19971–19976.
16. Roehle, A., K.P. Hoefig, D. Repsilber, *et al.* 2008. MicroRNA signatures characterize diffuse large B-cell lymphomas and follicular lymphomas. *Br. J. Haematol.* **142:** 732–744.
17. Eis, P.S., W. Tam, L. Sun, *et al.* 2005. Accumulation of miR-155 and BIC RNA in human B cell lymphomas. *Proc. Natl. Acad. Sci. USA* **102:** 3627–3632.
18. Lawrie, C.H., S. Soneji, T. Marafioti, *et al.* 2007. MicroRNA expression distinguishes between germinal center B cell-like and activated B cell-like subtypes of diffuse large B cell lymphoma. *Int. J. Cancer.* **121:** 1156–1161.
19. Rosenwald, A., G. Wright, K. Leroy, *et al.* 2003. Molecular diagnosis of primary mediastinal B cell lymphoma identifies a clinically favorable subgroup of diffuse large B cell lymphoma related to Hodgkin lymphoma. *J. Exp. Med.* **198:** 851–862.
20. Navarro, A., A. Gaya, A. Martinez, *et al.* 2008. MicroRNA expression profiling in classic Hodgkin lymphoma. *Blood* **111:** 2825–2832.

21. Van Vlierberghe, P., A. De Weer, P. Mestdagh, *et al.* 2009. Comparison of miRNA profiles of microdissected Hodgkin/Reed-Sternberg cells and Hodgkin cell lines versus CD77+ B-cells reveals a distinct subset of differentially expressed miRNAs. *Br. J. Haematol.* **147:** 686–690.

22. Navarro, A., T. Diaz, A. Martinez, *et al.* 2009. Regulation of JAK2 by miR-135a: prognostic impact in classic Hodgkin lymphoma. *Blood* **114:** 2945–2951.

23. Fabbri, M., R. Spizzo & G.A. Calin. 2010. High-throughput profiling in the hematopoietic system. *Methods Mol. Biol.* **667:** 79–91.

24. Fabbri, M. 2010. miRNAs as molecular biomarkers of cancer. *Expert Rev. Mol. Diagn.* **10:** 435–444.

25. Calin, G.A., R. Garzon, A. Cimmino, *et al.* 2006. MicroRNAs and leukemias: how strong is the connection. *Leuk. Res.* **30:** 653–655.

26. Call, T.G., R.L. Phyliky, P. Noel, *et al.* 1994. Incidence of chronic lymphocytic leukemia in Olmsted County, Minnesota, 1935 through 1989, with emphasis on changes in initial stage at diagnosis. *Mayo Clin. Proc.* **69:** 323–328.

27. Chiorazzi, N., K.R. Rai & M. Ferrarini. 2005. Chronic lymphocytic leukemia. *N. Engl. J. Med.* **352:** 804–815.

28. Calin, G.A., C.D. Dumitru, M. Shimizu, *et al.* 2002. Frequent deletions and down-regulation of micro- RNA genes miR15 and miR16 at 13q14 in chronic lymphocytic leukemia. *Proc. Natl. Acad. Sci. USA* **99:** 15524–15529.

29. Cimmino, A., G.A. Calin, M. Fabbri, *et al.* 2005. miR-15 and miR-16 induce apoptosis by targeting BCL2. *Proc. Natl. Acad. Sci. USA* **102:** 13944–13949.

30. Calin, G.A., A. Cimmino, M. Fabbri, *et al.* 2008. MiR-15a and miR-16–1 cluster functions in human leukemia. *Proc. Natl. Acad. Sci. USA* **105:** 5166–5171.

31. Pekarsky, Y., N. Zanesi, R.I. Aqeilan & C.M. Croce. 2007. Animal models for chronic lymphocytic leukemia. *J. Cell Biochem.* **100:** 1109–1118.

32. Raveche, E.S. 1990. Possible immunoregulatory role for CD5 + B cells. *Clin. Immunol. Immunopathol.* **56:** 135–150.

33. Raveche, E.S., E. Salerno, B.J. Scaglione, *et al.* 2007. Abnormal microRNA-16 locus with synteny to human 13q14 linked to CLL in NZB mice. *Blood* **109:** 5079–5086.

34. Klein, U., M. Lia, M. Crespo, *et al.* 2010. The DLEU2/miR-15a/16–1 cluster controls B cell proliferation and its deletion leads to chronic lymphocytic leukemia. *Cancer Cell* **17:** 28–40.

35. Liu, Y., M. Corcoran, O. Rasool, *et al.* 1997. Cloning of two candidate tumor suppressor genes within a 10 kb region on chromosome 13q14, frequently deleted in chronic lymphocytic leukemia. *Oncogene* **15:** 2463–2473.

36. Migliazza, A., F. Bosch, H. Komatsu, *et al.* 2001. Nucleotide sequence, transcription map, and mutation analysis of the 13q14 chromosomal region deleted in B-cell chronic lymphocytic leukemia. *Blood* **97:** 2098–2104.

37. Salerno, E., B.J. Scaglione, F.D. Coffman, *et al.* 2009. Correcting miR-15a/16 genetic defect in New Zealand Black mouse model of CLL enhances drug sensitivity. *Mol. Cancer Ther.* **8:** 2684–2692.

38. He, L., J.M. Thomson, M.T. Hemann, *et al.* 2005. A microRNA polycistron as a potential human oncogene. *Nature* **435:** 828–833.

39. Ota, A., H. Tagawa, S. Karnan, *et al.* 2004. Identification and characterization of a novel gene, C13orf25, as a target for 13q31-q32 amplification in malignant lymphoma. *Cancer Res.* **64:** 3087–3095.

40. Xiao, C., L. Srinivasan, D.P. Calado, *et al.* 2008. Lymphoproliferative disease and autoimmunity in mice with increased miR-17–92 expression in lymphocytes. *Nat. Immunol.* **9:** 405–414.

41. Ventura, A., A.G. Young, M.M. Winslow, *et al.* 2008. Targeted deletion reveals essential and overlapping functions of the miR-17 through 92 family of miRNA clusters. *Cell* **132:** 875–886.

42. Olive, V., M.J. Bennett, J.C. Walker, *et al.* 2009. miR-19 is a key oncogenic component of mir-17–92. *Genes Dev.* **23:** 2839–2849.

43. Mu, P., Y.C. Han, D. Betel, *et al.* 2009. Genetic dissection of the miR-17~92 cluster of microRNAs in Myc-induced B-cell lymphomas. *Genes Dev.* **23:** 2806–2811.

44. Volinia, S., G.A. Calin, C.G. Liu, *et al.* 2006. A microRNA expression signature of human solid tumors defines cancer gene targets. *Proc. Natl. Acad. Sci. USA* **103:** 2257–2261.

45. Calin, G.A., C.M. Croce. 2007. Investigation of microRNA alterations in leukemias and lymphomas. *Methods Enzymol.* **427:** 193–213.

46. Marton, S., M.R. Garcia, C. Robello, *et al.* 2008. Small RNAs analysis in CLL reveals a deregulation of miRNA expression and novel miRNA candidates of putative relevance in CLL pathogenesis. *Leukemia* **22:** 330–338.

47. Metzler, M., M. Wilda, K. Busch, *et al.* 2004. High expression of precursor microRNA-155/BIC RNA in children with Burkitt lymphoma. *Genes Chromosomes Cancer* **39:** 167–169.

48. Kluiver, J., S. Poppema, D. de Jong, *et al.* 2005. BIC and miR-155 are highly expressed in Hodgkin, primary mediastinal and diffuse large B cell lymphomas. *J. Pathol.* **207:** 243–249.

49. Nie, K., M. Gomez, P. Landgraf, *et al.* 2008. MicroRNA-mediated down-regulation of PRDM1/Blimp-1 in Hodgkin/Reed-Sternberg cells: a potential pathogenetic lesion in Hodgkin lymphomas. *Am. J. Pathol.* **173:** 242–252.

50. Costinean, S., N. Zanesi, Y. Pekarsky, *et al.* 2006. Pre-B cell proliferation and lymphoblastic leukemia/high-grade lymphoma in E(mu)-miR155 transgenic mice. *Proc. Natl. Acad. Sci. USA* **103:** 7024–7029.

51. Costinean, S., S.K. Sandhu, I.M. Pedersen, *et al.* 2009. Src homology 2 domain-containing inositol-5-phosphatase and CCAAT enhancer-binding protein beta are targeted by miR-155 in B cells of Emicro-MiR-155 transgenic mice. *Blood* **114:** 1374–1382.

52. Thai, T.H., D.P. Calado, S. Casola, *et al.* 2007. Regulation of the germinal center response by microRNA-155. *Science* **316:** 604–608.

53. Rodriguez, A., E. Vigorito & S. Clare. 2007. Requirement of bic/microRNA-155 for normal immune function. *Science* **316:** 608–611.

54. Cummins, J.M., Y. He, R.J. Leary, *et al.* 2006. The colorectal microRNAome. *Proc. Natl. Acad. Sci. USA* **103:** 3687–3692.

55. Akao, Y., Y. Nakagawa & T. Naoe. 2007. MicroRNA-143 and -145 in colon cancer. *DNA Cell Biol.* **26:** 311–320.

56. Slaby, O., M. Svoboda, P. Fabian, *et al.* 2007. Altered expression of miR-21, miR-31, miR-143 and miR-145 is related to

clinicopathologic features of colorectal cancer. *Oncology* **72**: 397–402.

57. Lanza, G., M. Ferracin, R. Gafa, *et al.* 2007. mRNA/microRNA gene expression profile in microsatellite unstable colorectal cancer. *Mol. Cancer* **6**: 1–11.

58. Valeri, N., P. Gasparini, M. Fabbri, *et al.* 2010. Modulation of mismatch repair and genomic stability by miR-155. *Proc. Natl. Acad. Sci. USA* **107**: 6982–6987.

59. Chen, X., Y. Ba, L. Ma, *et al.* 2008. Characterization of microRNAs in serum: a novel class of biomarkers for diagnosis of cancer and other diseases. *Cell Res.* **18**: 997–1006.

60. Ng, E.K., W.W. Chong, H. Jin, *et al.* 2009. Differential expression of microRNAs in plasma of patients with colorectal cancer: a potential marker for colorectal cancer screening. *Gut* **58**: 1375–1381.

61. Bloomston, M., W.L. Frankel, F. Petrocca, *et al.* 2007. MicroRNA expression patterns to differentiate pancreatic adenocarcinoma from normal pancreas and chronic pancreatitis. *JAMA* **297**: 1901–1908.

62. Szafranska, A.E., T.S. Davison, J. John, *et al.* 2007. MicroRNA expression alterations are linked to tumorigenesis and nonneoplastic processes in pancreatic ductal adenocarcinoma. *Oncogene* **26**: 4442–4452.

63. Szafranska, A.E., M. Doleshal, H.S. Edmunds, *et al.* 2008. Analysis of microRNAs in pancreatic fine-needle aspirates can classify benign and malignant tissues. *Clin. Chem.* **54**: 1716–1724.

64. Giovannetti, E., N. Funel, G.J. Peters, *et al.* 2010. MicroRNA-21 in pancreatic cancer: correlation with clinical outcome and pharmacologic aspects underlying its role in the modulation of gemcitabine activity. *Cancer Res.* **70**: 4528–4538.

65. Hwang, J.H., J. Voortman, E. Giovannetti, *et al.* 2010. Identification of microRNA-21 as a biomarker for chemoresistance and clinical outcome following adjuvant therapy in resectable pancreatic cancer. *PLoS One.* **5**: 1–12.

66. Jemal, A., R. Siegel, J. Xu & E. Ward. 2010. Cancer Statistics 2010. *CA Cancer J. Clin.* **60**: 277–300.

67. Yanaihara, N., N. Caplen, E. Bowman, *et al.* 2006. Unique microRNA molecular profiles in lung cancer diagnosis and prognosis. *Cancer Cell.* **9**: 189–198.

68. Yu, S.L., H.Y. Chen, G.C. Chang, *et al.* 2008. MicroRNA signature predicts survival and relapse in lung cancer. *Cancer Cell.* **13**: 48–57.

69. Fabbri, M., R. Garzon, A. Cimmino, *et al.* 2007. MicroRNA-29 family reverts aberrant methylation in lung cancer by targeting DNA methyltransferases 3A and 3B. *Proc. Natl. Acad. Sci. USA* **104**: 15805–15810.

70. Garofalo, M., G. Di Leva, G. Romano, *et al.* 2009. miR-221&222 regulate TRAIL resistance and enhance tumorigenicity through PTEN and TIMP3 downregulation. *Cancer Cell.* **16**: 498–509.

71. Kumar, M.S., S.J. Erkeland, R.E. Pester, *et al.* 2008. Suppression of non-small cell lung tumor development by the let-7 microRNA family. *Proc. Natl. Acad. Sci. USA* **105**: 3903–3908.

72. Johnson, S.M., H. Grosshans, J. Shingara, *et al.* 2005. RAS is regulated by the let-7 microRNA family. *Cell.* **120**: 635–647.

73. Iorio, M.V., M. Ferracin, C.G. Liu, *et al.* 2005. MicroRNA gene expression deregulation in human breast cancer. *Cancer Res.* **65**: 7065–7070.

74. Spizzo, R., M.S. Nicoloso, L. Lupini, *et al.* 2010. miR-145 participates with TP53 in a death-promoting regulatory loop and targets estrogen receptor-alpha in human breast cancer cells. *Cell Death Differ.* **17**: 246–254.

75. Sachdeva, M. & Y.Y. Mo. 2010. MicroRNA-145 suppresses cell invasion and metastasis by directly targeting mucin 1. *Cancer Res.* **70**: 378–387.

76. Faraoni, I., F.R. Antoinetti, J. Cardone, *et al.* 2009. miR-155 gene: a typical multifactorial microRNA. *Biochem. Biophys. Acta.* **1792**: 497–505.

77. Kong, W., L. He, M. Coppola, *et al.* 2010. MicroRNA-155 regulates cell survival, growth, and chemosensitivity by targeting FOXO3a in breast cancer. *J. Biol. Chem.* **285**: 17869–17879.

78. Jiang, S., H.W. Zhang, M.H. Lu, *et al.* 2010. MicroRNA-155 functions as an OncomiR in breast cancer by targeting the suppressor of cytokine signaling 1 gene. *Cancer Res.* **70**: 3119–3127.

79. Volinia, S., M. Galasso, S. Costinean, *et al.* 2010. Reprogramming of miRNA networks in cancer and leukemia. *Genome Res.* **20**: 589–599.

Ann. N.Y. Acad. Sci. ISSN 0077-8923

ANNALS OF THE NEW YORK ACADEMY OF SCIENCES

Issue: *Toward Personalized Medicine for Cancer*

From genomic landscapes to personalized cancer management—is there a roadmap?

Charles Swanton[1,2] and Carlos Caldas[3,4]

[1]Translational Cancer Therapeutics Laboratory, Cancer Research UK London Research Institute, London, United Kingdom. [2]Royal Marsden Hospital, Department of Medicine, Breast Unit, Sutton, United Kingdom. [3]Department of Oncology, University of Cambridge, Li Ka Shing Centre, Cambridge, United Kingdom. [4]Breast Cancer Functional Genomics Laboratory, Cancer Research UK Cambridge Research Institute, Cambridge, United Kingdom

Address for correspondence: Charles Swanton, Translational Cancer Therapeutics Laboratory, Cancer Research UK London Research Institute, London, United Kingdom. charles.swanton@cancer.org.uk

Despite rapid progress in annotating the human genome, progress in biomarker discovery has been limited, in part, due to the restricted adoption of biomarker analysis in clinical trials. In this short review we present a roadmap to drive progress in the field of personalized cancer management and patient stratification. We suggest that improved understanding of disease biology and drug response in advance of clinical trial design would enable novel biomarkers to be identified and prospectively evaluated during early phase trials; there will also be value in banked material from completed clinical trials to identify and validate biomarkers. Such progress requires standardized tissue collection protocols, novel bioinformatics strategies integrated with functional genomics analysis, and next generation sequencing technologies. We argue that the failure to adopt these methods rapidly into clinical trial design will increase late stage drug attrition, waste trial resources, and risk patient harm within unselected cohorts.

Keywords: drug resistance; predictive biomarker; prognostic biomarker; cancer management; clinical trial

Introduction

Progress in our understanding of cancer biology has accelerated dramatically over the last decade, driven for the most part by technological developments in molecular medicine. Advances in DNA copy number, gene expression, and next generation sequencing technologies have resulted in improved classification of solid tumors and provided insight into cancer genome complexity and heterogeneity.[1] Undoubtedly, progress in this field has influenced patient care in a positive way. Tumors such as non–small-cell lung cancer with epidermal growth factor receptor (EGFR) somatic mutations, human epidermal growth factor receptor 2 (Her-2)-positive breast cancer, gastrointestinal stromal tumors, chronic myeloid leukemia and Kirsten-Ras (KRAS) wild-type colorectal cancer, for which treatment options were limited fifteen years ago, now have therapeutics that offer tangible benefit in defined patient populations. The presence of a well-characterized predictive biomarker and a drug that is dependent on the biomarker for activity unites these diverse tumors, providing benchmarks against which further developments in cancer care will be measured.

Much has been learned from this process that can guide future developments in this field. First, failure to identify the predictive biomarker in advance of clinical trial design can lead to a roadblock in the drug development pathway and risk early drug attrition. Second, diseases such as renal cancer and metastatic melanoma, for which many medical oncologists had become despondent, are now becoming increasingly vulnerable to the new generation of targeted therapeutics, in part driven by an improved understanding of disease biology. Third, poor clinical trial design, poor tissue collection, and SOPs for tissue processing and a failure to develop parallel laboratory and clinical research strategies can seriously delay the identification of molecular mechanisms predictive of drug response. Fourth, failure to identify defined patient cohorts sensitive to a particular therapeutic, in a health–economic

doi: 10.1111/j.1749-6632.2010.05776.x

conscious climate, will impede health technology appraisal committee approval and the adoption of novel therapeutics into clinical practice. Finally, routine incorporation in early phase clinical trials of tumor pharmacodynamic and pharmacokinetic endpoints to identify the biologically active dose as well as the maximum tolerated dose will ensure that if efficacy is not seen, it is unlikely to be due to lack of target modulation.[2]

Adaptations to clinical trial design and the challenges of early phase clinical trial drug development are beyond the scope of this manuscript (succinctly reviewed in Ref. 2). In this review, we focus on developments in the field where lessons can be learned and suggest a biologically driven roadmap to avoid past obstacles while establishing key areas required for progress in the field.

Progress in biomarker development

A biomarker is any molecular "barcode" that may be obtained by analysis of mRNA, DNA, protein, or circulating tumor cells (CTC) or tumor-derived nucleic acids that may be used to stratify patients for treatment benefit within clinical trials, prognosticate patient outcome, or predict and/or monitor response to therapy.[3] In general, the goal of biomarker discovery is to identify which patient group to treat and which distinct therapeutic modality to offer that will result in improved outcome compared to no treatment or standard of care. Increasingly, selective biomarkers are being employed to refine tumor classification into homogeneous disease subtypes with more predictable outcomes within clinical trials, with treatment stratification biomarkers used to assess the impact of defined molecular changes upon therapeutic response.[3]

The requirement for more robust predictive and prognostic biomarkers is clearly illustrated in the management of primary breast cancer. Whilst impressive improvements in overall survival have been witnessed over the last 40 years across several tumor types including breast cancer,[4] undoubtedly clinicians are treating two cohorts of patients with systemic adjuvant therapy who will not benefit from treatment; the first cohort includes patients who have been cured by early diagnosis and optimal surgery with or without locoregional radiotherapy. This cohort is subject to overtreatment in the absence of prognostic biomarkers. A major step forward in this regard is the recent implementation of the stratification-based formalin-fixed, paraffin-embedded (FFPE) tissue quantitative polymerase chain reaction (qPCR) recurrence score in estrogen receptor positive early breast cancer to better define those at high risk of relapse who may preferentially be considered for chemotherapy in addition to tamoxifen.[5,6] A second group of patients will harbor intrinsic drug resistant disease, deriving no benefit from conventional treatment approaches. Identification of predictive biomarkers to conventional cytotoxics and novel targeted therapeutics is thus essential to optimally stratify patients for the appropriate treatment in order to identify which patients do not need further therapy and which patients should be considered for novel strategies within clinical trials.

Predictive biomarkers can be classified into three groups: cytotoxic, targeted, and molecular pathway directed.[1] Disappointingly, despite the fact that cytotoxic chemotherapy remains the mainstay of solid and hematological treatment approaches, predictive biomarkers of response to conventional cytotoxics are perhaps the least well characterized despite intensive investigation. The biomarker may represent the drug target itself, such as HER2 and trastuzumab response, estrogen receptor and benefit from tamoxifen, or EGFR somatic mutation status and response to EGFR tyrosine kinase inhibitors.

Advances in medium–high throughput genomics platforms have resulted in the rapid identification of tumor somatic mutations such as KRAS, EGFR, and the estimation of gene expression modules stratifying patient risk of relapse. Developments are set to accelerate with next generation sequencing technologies showing promise in the field of biomarker discovery. Recently, a technique called personalized analysis of rearranged ends was able to identify novel translocations in breast and colorectal cancer that could then be verified using PCR to detect these translocations in plasma DNA.[7] Such techniques have the potential to improve the detection of residual disease at surgical margins and, through the assessment of circulating tumor DNA (ctDNA), monitor response to chemotherapy or radiotherapy.

Pathway-driven therapeutics

Progress in the development of targeted therapeutics and their companion biomarkers has begun to challenge clinical practice and the management of solid tumors according to tumor type. It is becoming increasingly clear that tumors use similar mechanisms and signaling pathways in the transformation process that cross boundaries of tumor type and that molecular pathway directed therapeutics may play an increasingly important role in cancer management.[1] For example, the HER2 receptor, a commonly amplified or overexpressed gene in breast cancer, is also overexpressed or amplified in gastric cancer. Accordingly, patients with HER2 overexpressing or amplified gastric cancer derive a survival benefit from trastuzumab in combination with chemotherapy compared to chemotherapy alone.[8] Oncogenic KIT mutations, identified in gastrointestinal stromal tumors that are sensitive to imatinib,[9] are also present in a subset of mucosal and acral melanomas. It is becoming increasingly clear from case reports that melanomas harboring KIT mutations are also sensitive to imatinib.[10] The latter example illustrates an important concept. Determining drug efficacy in rare tumor types for which somatic drug-sensitising mutations occur at low frequency may increasingly rely on prospective case-report series to determine drug activity, challenging current drug approval strategies.

Accordingly, a future can be envisioned with the costs of genomic approaches declining rapidly, where patients presenting in the clinical setting may have their tumor biopsied and cancer genome and transcriptome sequenced in order to identify panels of potential driver mutations for which targeted therapeutics exist.

Molecular understanding of drug response is central to biomarker discovery

The clinical development of gefitinib illustrates the importance of biomarker development in advance of clinical trial design. Failure to identify a robust biomarker can result in drug development delays and even result in clinical harm through the treatment of a biomarker negative cohort who may actually have a poorer outcome with a new therapeutic compared to standard of care.

EGFR was first identified in the early 1980s as an oncogene-encoded protein by Downward and colleagues, who described six peptides derived from the human epidermal growth factor receptor with close similarity to viral avian erythroblastosis oncogene B (v-erb-B) transforming protein of avian erthryoblastosis virus[11] and the receptor's auto-

phosphorylation and activation following receptor–ligand engagement.[12] The introduction of the small molecule inhibitor of EGFR, gefitinib, into clinical trials resulted in evidence of single agent activity (9–12% partial response rates) in patients with stage IIIB/IV pretreated NSCLC.[13] At this stage in the drug development strategy, there was no means of identifying the responding population or a predictive biomarker to use in subsequent trials. Twenty years following the identification of the EGFR receptor, two large phase III trials of gefitinib in combination with first line chemotherapy in non-small cell lung cancer (NSCLC) (INTACT 1 [Iressa Non-small cell lung cancer Trial Assessing Combination Treatment], and INTACT 2) failed to demonstrate improved efficacy over chemotherapy alone.[14] The authors acknowledged that establishing the reasons for this failure required more preclinical testing. A rational basis for drug response was published by Lynch and colleagues, who determined that patients with gefitinib sensitive NSCLC harbored somatic mutations in the tyrosine kinase domain of EGFR, which rendered the receptor more biologically active and sensitive to gefitinib in vitro.[15] Finally, 25 years after the receptor was first identified, Mok and colleagues demonstrated that gefitinib has superior efficacy compared to carboplatin/paclitaxel as a first line treatment in non-smokers and the presence of a somatic EGFR tyrosine kinase domain mutation could serve as a robust predictive biomarker.[16] Perhaps the most salient result of this analysis is that patients without a somatic EGFR tyrosine kinase domain mutation had a poorer outcome when treated with gefitinib compared to standard of care chemotherapy, indicating that failure to address biomarker requirements can result in patient harm.

The recognition that drug target biology may be extremely complex is vital to appropriate biomarker identification and patient selection to minimize the risk of patient harm and maximize therapeutic benefit. Recently, Marais and colleagues provided evidence that BRAF inhibition of kinase dead BRAF in the presence of oncogenic RAS can drive the association of V-RAF-1 murine leukemia viral oncogene homolog 1 (CRAF) with V-RAF murine sarcoma viral oncogene homolog B1 (BRAF), resulting in CRAF-mediated mitogen-activated protein kinase/ERK kinase (MEK)/extracellular signal-regulated kinase (ERK) pathway activation and the initiation of tumorigenesis.[17] As the authors suggest, such studies raise serious concerns regarding the treatment of patients with BRAF selective inhibitors in the presence of tumor oncogenic RAS mutations. Such studies, focusing on cell signaling networks that influence drug response, illustrate their requirement for the identification of patient cohorts who should not be treated with specific pathway inhibitors, and suggest future combinatorial approaches to minimize the emergence of drug resistant clones. These approaches also illustrate that a predictive biomarker may not rely on the clinical assessment of one candidate but may depend on the parallel identification of mutations in upstream or downstream pathway regulators.

Despite clear evidence that the parallel development of the molecular understanding of drug response to accelerate predictive biomarker discovery is of vital importance for the success of a targeted therapeutic, there are still many examples of agents with activity in a minority of patients. There is still no definition as to how this sensitive patient cohort should be identified.

Toward a roadmap for personalized cancer treatment

Integrating functional with tumor genomics to support biomarker discovery

In order to attempt to identify molecular regulators of drug response and sensitivity, genome wide analytical techniques incorporating gene expression or DNA copy number have been employed with the capacity to generate excessive quantities of data relative to the number of patients in the cohort. Such associative learning studies, gleaned through the analysis of multiple genomics parameters from only a handful of patients whilst documenting gene sets that correlate with a particular clinical parameter such as drug response, are rarely concordant when studying the same parameter across multiple studies.[18]

An alternative and perhaps more logical approach is to identify relevant genomic predictors in advance of, or in parallel with clinical trial tumor analysis (Fig. 1). Such an approach aims to reduce the number of candidate genes associated with drug response to those functionally implicated in altering drug sensitivity thereby minimizing the number of potentially testable hypotheses. RNA interference screening techniques are now readily applicable to the analysis of drug resistance pathways and to identify synthetic lethal interactions on prespecified genetic backgrounds.[19–21] Several groups have now published evidence that RNA interference approaches can be used to identify relevant predictors of drug response from retrospective patient cohort or clinical trial analyses. In a large-scale screen to identify mediators of trastuzumab response, phosphatase and tensin homolog (PTEN) loss was the only gene identified, indicating a major role for the Phosphatidylinositol 3-kinase-V-AKT murine thymoma viral oncogene homolog 1 (PI3K-AKT) signaling pathway.[22] Follow-up analysis in a small cohort of 55 breast cancer patients revealed that a low PTEN expression or PIK3CA mutation status was associated with poorer outcome following trastuzumab therapy. In a similar manner, Iorns and colleagues identified the silencing of cyclin dependent kinase 10 (CDK10) contributed to tamoxifen resistance in an RNA interference screen of the human kinome.[23] In follow up analysis of two clinical datasets of 87 and 38 breast cancer patients treated with adjuvant Tamoxifen, low CDK10 mRNA expression was associated with significantly poorer outcome in both datasets.

Using similar RNA interference screening approaches, we have identified several genes involved in mitotic arrest and ceramide metabolism that promote resistance to paclitaxel when silenced in three cancer cell lines.[24] Expression of a "functional metagene" comprising mitotic arrest and ceramide pathway genes that consistently influenced paclitaxel sensitivity across three cancer cell lines of different tumor origin was found to be predictive of paclitaxel-specific pathological complete response (pCR) in a retrospective analysis of two breast cancer clinical trials of paclitaxel/5-fluorouracil, adriamycin and cyclophosphamide (FAC) regimens (n = 233 patients). Since the RNAi screen specifically addressed mediators of drug response in an estrogen receptor (ER) negative/ERBB2 negative cancer cell-line, we addressed the power of the metagene to predict pCR in this subtype and was found to be significantly predictive of response in this subtype in multivariate analysis.[25]

In this RNA interference (RNAi) drug resistance screen, we noted several genes that promoted paclitaxel resistance when silenced also initiated aneuploidy independent of drug exposure, leading to the hypothesis that molecular pathways monitoring

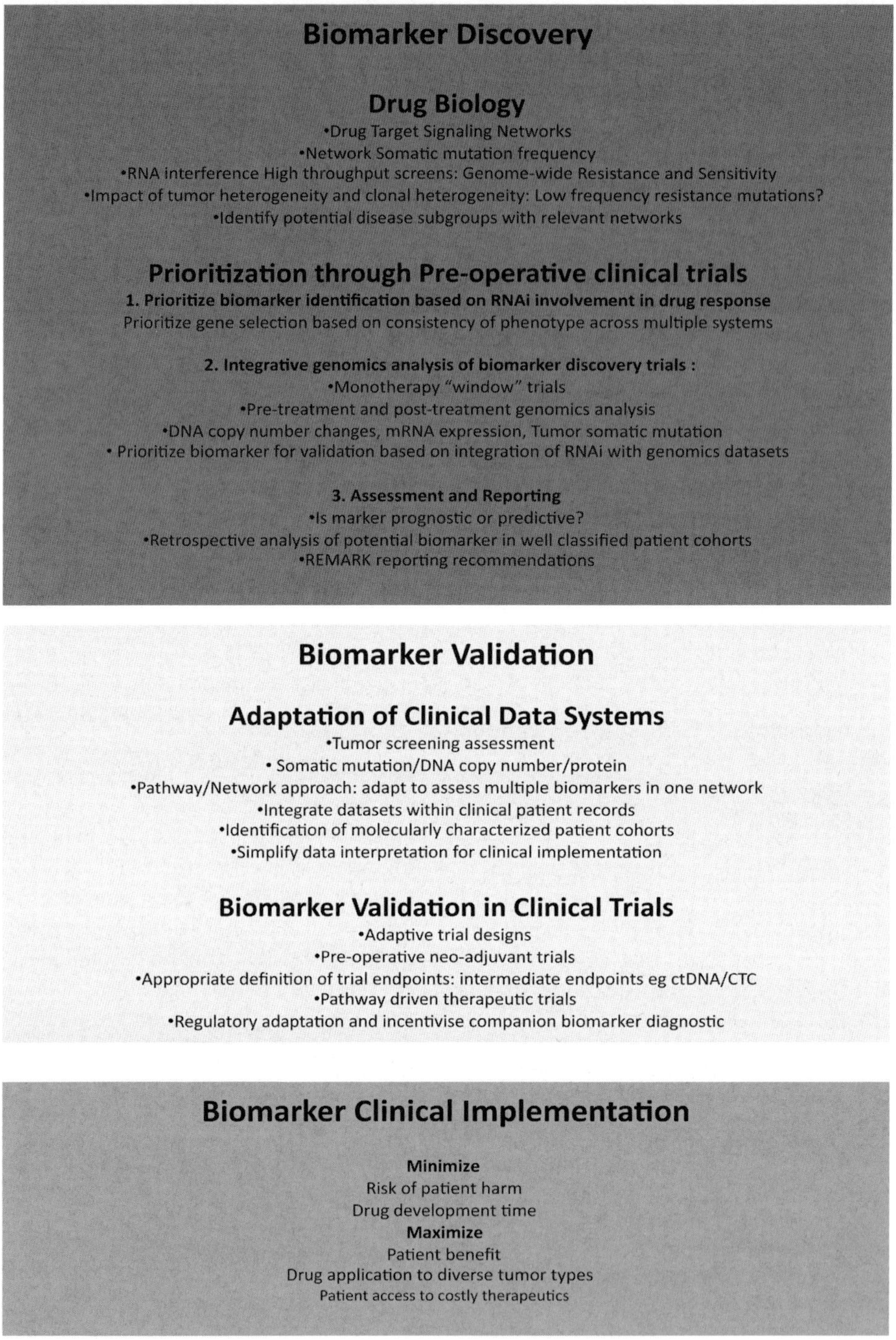

Biomarker Discovery

Drug Biology
•Drug Target Signaling Networks
•Network Somatic mutation frequency
•RNA interference High throughput screens: Genome-wide Resistance and Sensitivity
•Impact of tumor heterogeneity and clonal heterogeneity: Low frequency resistance mutations?
•Identify potential disease subgroups with relevant networks

Prioritization through Pre-operative clinical trials
1. Prioritize biomarker identification based on RNAi involvement in drug response
Prioritize gene selection based on consistency of phenotype across multiple systems

2. Integrative genomics analysis of biomarker discovery trials :
•Monotherapy "window" trials
•Pre-treatment and post-treatment genomics analysis
•DNA copy number changes, mRNA expression, Tumor somatic mutation
• Prioritize biomarker for validation based on integration of RNAi with genomics datasets

3. Assessment and Reporting
•Is marker prognostic or predictive?
•Retrospective analysis of potential biomarker in well classified patient cohorts
•REMARK reporting recommendations

Biomarker Validation

Adaptation of Clinical Data Systems
•Tumor screening assessment
• Somatic mutation/DNA copy number/protein
•Pathway/Network approach: adapt to assess multiple biomarkers in one network
•Integrate datasets within clinical patient records
•Identification of molecularly characterized patient cohorts
•Simplify data interpretation for clinical implementation

Biomarker Validation in Clinical Trials
•Adaptive trial designs
•Pre-operative neo-adjuvant trials
•Appropriate definition of trial endpoints: intermediate endpoints eg ctDNA/CTC
•Pathway driven therapeutic trials
•Regulatory adaptation and incentivise companion biomarker diagnostic

Biomarker Clinical Implementation

Minimize
Risk of patient harm
Drug development time
Maximize
Patient benefit
Drug application to diverse tumor types
Patient access to costly therapeutics

Figure 1. RNA interference screening techniques are now readily applicable to the analysis of drug resistance pathways and to identify synthetic lethal interactions on prespecified genetic backgrounds.

chromosomal stability might impact upon those regulating paclitaxel response. Consistent with this observation, chromosomal instability, as measured by the chromosomal instability 70 gene signature (CIN70) expression signature, was associated with primary paclitaxel resistance in the OV01 ovarian cancer clinical trial in which 40 patients were randomized to either paclitaxel or carboplatin chemotherapy prior to surgery.[26]

These studies take a similar approach. First, they derive a high stringency candidate list of validated genes impacting upon drug response *in vitro* and test for their association with clinical outcome in retrospective analysis of clinical cohorts. Through the limitation of the number of genes tested, functionally implicated in drug response, the number of potential testable hypotheses is restricted, which may reduce the risk of false positive conclusions driven by multiple testing flaws in earlier gene expression association studies. Strikingly, all of these studies have one aspect in common, their validation in small molecularly defined retrospective patient cohorts, indicating that if the biology of drug response is well understood from laboratory studies, large phase II/III trial cohorts may not be required to demonstrate an association of a putative biomarker with drug response in appropriately molecularly characterized patients.

Retrospective analysis of clinical genomics datasets

Implementation of retrospective subgroup analyses has proven valuable in defining distinct patient subgroups that benefit preferentially from targeted therapeutic approaches. Examples include EGFR monoclonal antibody therapy benefit and KRAS wild type status,[27] HER2 status and paclitaxel benefit,[28] and EGFR mutation status and gefitinib survival benefit.[29]

Increasingly, the molecular annotation of the cancer genome across diverse tumor types has led to a vast amount of publicly available gene expression and DNA copy number analyses that allow hypotheses derived from laboratory studies to be challenged retrospectively in clinical datasets, which may incorporate meta-analysis techniques. Retrospective analyses have proven useful for several functional genomics RNA interference strategies in order to define the relevance of a putative biomarker

to treatment response in defined breast cancer subtypes.[22,23,25]

Histopathologically, identical tumors may have different outcomes irrespective of treatment that are governed by subtle molecular changes.[30] Novel markers that enable the distinction of two previously identical tumors by routine pathology may distinguish tumor subtypes with different clinical outcomes. Meta-analysis approaches through the combination of diverse clinical datasets have the power to identify consistent prognostic differences within specific disease subtypes. For example, in a meta-analysis of 10,000 breast cancers, Blows and colleagues recently determined the prognostic relevance of six subtypes of breast cancer defined by expression of immunohistochemical markers (ER, PR [progesterone receptor], ERBB2 [avian erythroblastosis oncogene B2], CK5 [cytokeratin], CK6, and EGFR),[31] formally demonstrating that each subtype has a different relationship between hazard ratio for relapse with time that is independent of adjuvant therapy. Retrospective molecular analyses of clinical trial tissue datasets can prove fruitful in determining the predictive relevance of previously defined molecular aberrations, such as the importance of chromosome 17 centromeric enumeration probe duplication and anthracycline benefit in the adjuvant therapy of primary breast cancer.[32]

Identification of distinct disease subtypes, each with different clinical outcomes that are independent of treatment through such retrospective analyses, are essential for appropriate stratification methods when designing clinical trials to examine predictive biomarker validity. Such considerations will avoid false conclusions regarding drug efficacy in a disease subtype that would have had a favorable outcome regardless of treatment.

Parallel development of clinical trial– and functional genomics–driven biomarker discovery

The approach taken by a European Union consortium, Personalized RNA interference to Enhance the Delivery of Individualized Chemotherapeutics and Targeted therapies (PREDICT), is to take extend these efforts in parallel with drug development within clinical trials in a prospective manner. This consortium is using a combination of genome wide RNA interference drug resistance screening approaches to address response to mammalian target of rapamycin (mTOR) and multi-targeted tyrosine kinase inhibitors used in clinical practice, for which no robust predictive biomarkers exist.

This consortium sets out to define a roadmap through which developments in the genomic characterization of human tumors treated within clinical trials with well defined operating procedures for tissue collection can be used to identify the next generation of biomarkers. The consortium will use techniques such as next generation exome sequencing technologies, whole genome single nucleotide polymorphism/comparative genomic hybridisation (SNP/CGH), and mRNA expression analysis of tumors treated within clinical trials with defined response assessment. Data from these assessments will be integrated in parallel with *in vitro* RNA interference screening techniques to identify genes functionally implicated in drug response *in vivo* in discovery clinical trial cohorts. A high stringency short list of genes that are subject to altered expression, copy number change, or somatic mutation, selected from a validated list of genes that have shown to consistently alter drug response from unbiased whole genome RNAi screens *in vitro* across multiple cancer cell line systems, will be interrogated in subsequent trial validation cohorts.

Adaptive trial designs to validate a biomarker

Recent cancer genome sequencing studies using next-generation sequencing technologies in breast cancer have shed light on the extent of somatic mutational heterogeneity between patients with tumors of the same histopathological classification.[33–35] In the most extensive study, Stephens and colleagues identified that none of the fusion genes identified in 14 breast cancers and breast cancer cell lines were shared between tumors and three in-frame fusions were not present in 288 other tumors analyzed. These data begin to indicate that there are likely to be multiple genomic rearrangements and somatic mutations present in each tumor that are not shared at high frequency between patients. In a further study, Navin and colleagues explored breast cancer heterogeneity within the same tumor using a technique called sector-ploidy profiling.[36] They identified several examples of intra-tumoral heterogeneity in ploidy status or genomic aberrations. Conceivably, such intra-tumoral heterogeneity may impact upon tumor sampling error for biomarker identification. This inter- and intra-tumoral hetero-

geneity may present extreme challenges in terms of cost and time for biomarker directed clinical trials with targeted therapeutics in small highly selected patient cohorts.

The profound inter-tumoral heterogeneity identified in cancer genome sequencing studies and the fact that a potential biomarker of drug response may be present in a small proportion of patients has precipitated changes to clinical trial design to adapt to the challenges of personalized medicine approaches in cases where the biomarker may be present at a low frequency patient cohorts.

Adaptive clinical trial designs are likely to be a vital component of drug development for multiple targeted therapeutics. Such designs, exemplified by I-SPY2 (Investigation of Serial Studies to Predict Your Therapeutic Response with Imaging And moLecular Analysis 2) and BATTLE (Biomarker-integrated Approaches of Targeted Therapy for Lung Cancer Elimination), allow researchers to review data during the clinical trial and adapt patient recruitment accordingly. Depending on early response assessment, such trials might allow researchers to test multiple potential biomarker selected patient cohorts for different therapeutic approaches and prioritize patients for distinct arms of the trial.

Such trial designs require robust and advanced statistical techniques and may heighten the risk of false positive conclusions. Particular care must be given to determining whether a putative predictive biomarker may also have prognostic relevance, where patient cohorts may have a superior outcome determined by the biomarker used to select them rather than the systemic therapy itself. Because of the requirement for interim analyses and clinician unblinding, traditional trial double-blind standards may be affected.[37]

Trial endpoints

Traditional clinical trial endpoints, such as progression free or overall survival, may require adaptation to the myriad of different small molecule inhibitors in clinical development in order to adapt studies to the therapeutic in question, accelerate the drug development process, and attempt to maximize patient benefit. Endpoints used to assess cytotoxics early in the drug development process, such as tumor imaging response defined by RECIST (Response Evaluation Criteria for Solid Tumors), may be less relevant to targeted therapeutics predicted to have a cytostatic rather than cytotoxic impact on tumor growth.

Increasingly, approaches using circulating blood borne markers representative of disease activity, such as CTC and ctDNA, are being considered for integration within clinical trials as intermediate endpoint biomarkers of outcome.[2]

Biomarker reporting

Once a biomarker is identified that might predict patient prognosis or response to therapy, further elaborate assessments are required to validate its use in patient cohorts, assess inter- and intra-laboratory reproducibility of the assay and estimate the impact of intra-tumoral heterogeneity on the presence of the biomarker in tumor samples. Recently, key recommendations were proposed for the reporting of prognostic markers to enable others to assess the validity of the methodologies and conclusions drawn from each study. Recommendations from this work included the description of prespecified hypotheses, including statistical power analyses, description of the patient cohorts in terms of tumor histopathological and stage characteristics and treatments received with clinical endpoints, and detailed assay protocols enabling data reproducibility and the relationship of the marker to standard prognostic variables to be confirmed.[38]

Roadmap challenges

Biomarker incentivization and adoption

Despite impressive advances in our ability to annotate the cancer genome both descriptively and functionally, attempts to identify validated predictive biomarkers have been disappointing. From an industry perspective, predictive biomarkers have the capacity to restrict market-share, yet from a health technology appraisal perspective, identification of predictive biomarkers are vital to reduce drug expenditure and improve patient quality of life.[39,40] However, adversity can be turned to advantage, since through a better understanding of drug response and molecular characterization of tumors, a drug with activity in one tumor type can be expanded for use in another in a pathway-driven therapeutic approach.[41]

In the future, with increasing health economics pressures, drug approval is likely to be enhanced and clinical adoption maximized if companion diagnostics are fully integrated with drug development. Nevertheless, it is recognized that there are regulatory hurdles to consider during companion biomarker diagnostic development, as both drug and biomarker have to meet strict regulatory thresholds for marketing approval and implementation within the clinical setting (reviewed in [39]). Such a complex and costly regulatory process is likely to prove a major disincentive towards the implementation of personalized therapeutics, prompting some to suggest that flexibility should be built into biomarker validation during the postmarketing period to fully clarify that patients whose tumors are not defined as biomarker positive derive no benefit from therapy.

There is also a major disparity in the number of unique biomarkers in each tumor type used to select patients for clinical trials. In a recent review of phase III trials, Sikorski and Yao identified a major disparity in biomarker adoption across tumor types relative to their frequency of occurrence.[3] The conclusion from these data is that rarer diseases, such as leukemia, are being fragmented into increasingly rare disease subtypes, whilst a common disease, such as prostate cancer, has only one selection marker, prostate-specific antigen (PSA), used in clinical trial development. The authors suggest that this may reflect the ease with which markers can be identified (cluster of differentiation [CD] antigens from peripheral blood) and patients selected in hematological malignancies and their translocation-driven nature. A recurring theme amongst solid tumors is the molecular heterogeneity both between patients (inter-tumor heterogeneity) and at the individual tumor level (intra-tumor heterogeneity) that may impede identification of prognosis-relevant biomarkers. Such observations emphasize the importance of retrospective annotation of disease biology and outcome in complex heterogeneous disease types using whole genome next generation sequencing technologies, through such consortia as the Cancer Genome Project and related networks.[42]

Tumor heterogeneity

Our current understanding of heterogeneity within individual tumors is relatively rudimentary, resulting from the lack of robust techniques to address cell-to-cell variation in tumor samples. Such heterogeneity is likely to be critical to the acquisition of drug resistance, as has recently been demonstrated by the Settleman laboratory[43]; the authors detected a low frequency population of drug-resistant cells with insulin-like growth factor 1 (IGF1) signaling pathway activity and chromatin alterations driven by a histone demethylase Jarid1A. The acquisition of this altered state is transient and reversible, enabling the acquisition of drug resistance driven by phenotypic heterogeneity. Similarly, Turke and colleagues have explored cancer cell phenotypic heterogeneity as a contributor to EGFR inhibitor resistance. Amplification of met proto-oncogene (MET) is observed in approximately 20% of tumors that have acquired resistance to EGFR tyrosine kinase inhibitors,[44] and in this study, low frequency populations of cancer cells, accounting for <1% of the tumor cells, with MET amplification prior to drug exposure were identified.[45]

Intra-tumor heterogeneity has recently been studied using DNA copy number approaches from regional sections of breast carcinomas to assess structural chromosomal instability (sector-ploidy profiling). Eleven of twenty breast cancers studied displayed evidence of different genomic alterations within the same tumor. Numerical chromosome instability (driven by whole chromosome mis-segregation events at mitosis) can also contribute to intra-tumoral heterogeneity. Breast cancer analyses indicate that numerical chromosomal instability (referred to as unstable aneuploidy or clone heterogeneity) occurs in 33–53% of invasive breast cancers (21/63, 9/20, and 55/104 breast carcinoma samples[46–48]). Intra-tumoral heterogeneity may result in at least two disturbing implications. First, tumor sampling error may lead to false negative conclusions concerning biomarker prevalence.[40] Second, elegant mouse tumor models suggest that numerical chromosomal heterogeneity may result in early tumor relapse after therapeutic intervention.[49]

Such low frequency genetic and epigenetic events occurring within tumor subpopulations that have the capacity to alter clinical outcome and that might be difficult to detect prior to drug exposure have major implications in the assessment and implementation of a biomarker into clinical practice. This event emphasizes the need to understand intrinsic cellular pathways regulating drug response to maximize the potential for combination strategies to delay the acquisition of resistance.

Are clinically applicable predictive biomarkers necessarily identifiable?

Next generation sequencing analysis of solid tumors has revealed the extraordinary complexity of the mutational landscape both in terms of gross chromosomal rearrangements and somatic mutations, with several "driver" genes identifiable within individual tumors, few of which are shared between patients.[33–35,50,51]

Researchers have attempted to define order from a seemingly chaotic mutational spectrum, with observations that somatic mutations often occur within amplified or deleted genomic regions or within pathway networks.[50] The anticipation is that such networks may be targetable at nodal points despite their peturbation by diverse low frequency somatic events. Even if all major molecular regulators of a network can be identified, developing validated clinical assays capable of assessing multiple somatic events to identify those tumors, most likely to display network disruption, is likely to impose major clinical challenges, both in terms of cost and time. For such a process to become feasible, major modifications are likely to be required in terms of clinical practice, tumor tissue collection SOPs, and the adaptation of clinical data systems to allow clinicians to rapidly interpret and access genomics datasets to define the optimal individualized treatment strategy. Such endeavors, when considered in parallel with the compounded impact of low frequency events, driven by tumor clonal heterogeneity, tumor sampling error, biomarker assay reproducibility, complexity of tumor:stroma interactions, and adaptations during therapy together with the regulatory hurdles required for biomarker implementation, pose serious challenges for future developments in patient stratification.

Conclusions

There are clear ethical and health economic considerations to re-address the way in which therapeutic agents are used in oncology practice. Deficiencies in our understanding of drug response pathways have led to notable failures in drug development strategies that can lead to patient harm in biomarker negative cohorts. Thus, clearer strategies to define pathways predictive of tumor drug sensitivity pathways in advance of trial design are essential to minimize risk to patients and maximize clinical trial resource and patient benefit. If consistent biomarkers of drug response are identifiable, then a logical approach to clinical trial design and tumor tissue analysis to include whole genome exon sequencing analysis combined with RNA interference functional genomics analysis may provide a rational strategy. Even with such approaches, significant adaptations to regulatory approval pathways, clinical data systems, biomarker assay development to include multiple network parameters, and a deeper understanding of tumor clonal heterogeneity will be required to fully realize the potential of patient stratification and personalized therapeutics.

Conflicts of Interest

The authors declare no conflicts of interest.

References

1. Swanton, C. & C. Caldas. 2009. Molecular classification of solid tumors: towards pathway-driven therapeutics. *Br. J. Cancer* **100:** 1517–1522.
2. Yap, T.A. *et al.* 2010. Envisioning the future of early anticancer drug development. *Nat. Rev. Cancer* **10:** 514–523.
3. Sikorski, R. & B. Yao 2010. Visualizing the landscape of selection biomarkers in current phase III oncology clinical trials. *Sci. Transl. Med.* **2:** 34ps27.
4. Jemal, A., E. Ward, & M. Thun. 2010. Declining death rates reflect progress against cancer. *PLoS One* **5:** e9584.
5. Paik, S. *et al.* 2004. A multigene assay to predict recurrence of tamoxifen-treated, node-negative breast cancer. *N. Engl. J. Med.* **351:** 2817–2826.
6. Paik, S. *et al.* 2006. Gene expression and benefit of chemotherapy in women with node-negative, estrogen receptor-positive breast cancer. *J. Clin. Oncol.* **24:** 3726–3734.
7. Leary, R.J. *et al.* 2010. Development of personalized tumor biomarkers using massively parallel sequencing. *Sci. Transl. Med.* **2:** 20ra14.
8. Van Cutsem, E. *et al.* 2009. Efficacy results from the ToGA trial: a phase III study of trastuzumab added to standard chemotherapy (CT) in first-line human epidermal growth factor receptor 2 (HER2)-positive advanced gastric cancer (GC). *J. Clin. Oncol.* **27:** 18s.
9. Heinrich, M.C. *et al.* 2006. Molecular correlates of imatinib resistance in gastrointestinal stromal tumors. *J. Clin. Oncol.* **24:** 4764–4774.
10. Handolias, D., *et al.* 2010. Clinical responses observed with imatinib or sorafenib in melanoma patients expressing mutations in KIT. *Br. J. Cancer* **102:** 1219–1223.
11. Downward, J. *et al.* 1984. Close similarity of epidermal growth factor receptor and v-erb-B oncogene protein sequences. *Nature* **307:** 521–527.
12. Downward, J., P. Parker, & M.D. Waterfield. 1984. Autophosphorylation sites on the epidermal growth factor receptor. *Nature* **311:** 483–485.
13. Kris, M.G. *et al.* 2003. Efficacy of gefitinib, an inhibitor of the epidermal growth factor receptor tyrosine kinase, in

symptomatic patients with non-small cell lung cancer: a randomized trial. *JAMA* **290:** 2149–2158.
14. Giaccone, G. *et al.* 2004. Gefitinib in combination with gemcitabine and cisplatin in advanced non-small-cell lung cancer: a phase III trial–INTACT 1. *J. Clin. Oncol.* **22:** 777–784.
15. Lynch, T.J. *et al.* 2004. Activating mutations in the epidermal growth factor receptor underlying responsiveness of non-small-cell lung cancer to gefitinib. *N. Engl. J. Med.* **350:** 2129–2139.
16. Mok, T.S. *et al.* 2009. Gefitinib or carboplatin-paclitaxel in pulmonary adenocarcinoma. *N. Engl. J. Med.* **361:** 947–957.
17. Heidorn, S.J. *et al.* 2010. Kinase-dead BRAF and oncogenic RAS cooperate to drive tumor progression through CRAF. *Cell* **140:** 209–221.
18. Ein-Dor, L., O. Zuk, & E. Domany. 2006. Thousands of samples are needed to generate a robust gene list for predicting outcome in cancer. *Proc. Natl. Acad. Sci. USA* **103:** 5923–5928.
19. Ashworth, A. 2008. A synthetic lethal therapeutic approach: poly(ADP) ribose polymerase inhibitors for the treatment of cancers deficient in DNA double-strand break repair. *J. Clin. Oncol.* **26:** 3785–3790.
20. Iorns, E. *et al.* 2007. Utilizing RNA interference to enhance cancer drug discovery. *Nat. Rev. Drug. Discov.* **6:** 556–568.
21. Swanton, C. *et al.* 2008. Functional genomic analysis of drug sensitivity pathways to guide adjuvant strategies in breast cancer. *Breast Cancer Res.* **10:** 214–221.
22. Berns, K. *et al.* 2007. A functional genetic approach identifies the PI3K pathway as a major determinant of trastuzumab resistance in breast cancer. *Cancer Cell* **12:** 395–402.
23. Iorns, E. *et al.* 2008. Identification of CDK10 as an important determinant of resistance to endocrine therapy for breast cancer. *Cancer Cell* **13:** 91–104.
24. Swanton, C. *et al.* 2007. Regulators of mitotic arrest and ceramide metabolism are determinants of sensitivity to paclitaxel and other chemotherapeutic drugs. *Cancer Cell* **11:** 498–512.
25. Juul, N. *et al.* 2010. Assessment of an RNA interference screen-derived mitotic and ceramide pathway metagene as a predictor of response to neoadjuvant paclitaxel for primary triple-negative breast cancer: a retrospective analysis of five clinical trials. *Lancet Oncol* **11:** 358–365.
26. Swanton, C. *et al.* 2009. Chromosomal instability determines taxane response. *Proc. Natl. Acad. Sci. USA* **106:** 8671–8676.
27. Amado, R.G. *et al.* 2008. Wild-type KRAS is required for panitumumab efficacy in patients with metastatic colorectal cancer. *J. Clin. Oncol.* **26:** 1626–1634.
28. Hayes, D.F. *et al.* 2007. HER2 and response to paclitaxel in node-positive breast cancer. *N. Engl. J. Med.* **357:** 1496–1506.
29. Takano, T. *et al.* 2008. EGFR mutations predict survival benefit from gefitinib in patients with advanced lung adenocarcinoma: a historical comparison of patients treated before and after gefitinib approval in Japan. *J. Clin. Oncol.* **26:** 5589–5595.
30. Mulligan, A.M. *et al.* 2008. Prognostic effect of basal-like breast cancers is time dependent: evidence from tissue microarray studies on a lymph node-negative cohort. *Clin. Cancer Res.* **14:** 4168–4174.

31. Blows, F.M. *et al.* 2010. Subtyping of breast cancer by immunohistochemistry to investigate a relationship between subtype and short and long term survival: a collaborative analysis of data for 10,159 cases from 12 studies. *PLoS Med.* **7:** e1000279.

32. Bartlett, J.M. *et al.* 2010. Predictive markers of anthracycline benefit: a prospectively planned analysis of the UK National Epirubicin Adjuvant Trial (NEAT/BR9601). *Lancet Oncol.* **11:** 266–274.

33. Shah, S.P. *et al.* 2009. Mutational evolution in a lobular breast tumor profiled at single nucleotide resolution. *Nature* **461:** 809–813.

34. Stephens, P.J. *et al.* 2009. Complex landscapes of somatic rearrangement in human breast cancer genomes. *Nature* **462:** 1005–1010.

35. Ding, L. *et al.* 2010. Genome remodelling in a basal-like breast cancer metastasis and xenograft. *Nature* **464:** 999–1005.

36. Navin, N. *et al.* 2010. Inferring tumor progression from genomic heterogeneity. *Genome Res.* **20:** 68–80.

37. 2010. Editorial: Time to adapt. *Nature* **464:** 1245–1246.

38. McShane, L.M. *et al.* 2005. Reporting recommendations for tumor MARKer prognostic studies (REMARK). *Br. J. Cancer* **93:** 387–391.

39. Schilsky, R.L. 2010. Personalized medicine in oncology: the future is now. *Nat. Rev. Drug Discov.* **9:** 363–366.

40. Tan, D.S. *et al.* 2010. Anti-cancer drug resistance; understanding the mechanisms through the use of integrative genomics and functional RNA interference. *Eur. J. Cancer* **46:** 2166–2177.

41. Bernards, R. 2010. It's diagnostics, stupid. *Cell* **141:** 13–17.

42. Hudson, T.J. *et al.* 2010. International network of cancer genome projects. *Nature* 464: 993–998.

43. Sharma, S.V. *et al.* 2010. A chromatin-mediated reversible drug-tolerant state in cancer cell subpopulations. *Cell* **141:** 69–80.

44. Bean, J. *et al.* 2007. MET amplification occurs with or without T790M mutations in EGFR mutant lung tumors with acquired resistance to gefitinib or erlotinib. *Proc. Natl. Acad. Sci. USA* **104:** 20932–20937.

45. Turke, A.B. *et al.* 2010. Preexistence and clonal selection of MET amplification in EGFR mutant NSCLC. *Cancer Cell* **17:** 77–88.

46. Farabegoli, F. *et al.* 2001. Clone heterogeneity in diploid and aneuploid breast carcinomas as detected by FISH. *Cytometry* **46:** 50–56.

47. Kronenwett, U. *et al.* 2004. Improved grading of breast adenocarcinomas based on genomic instability. *Cancer Res.* **64:** 904–909.

48. Lingle, W.L. *et al.* 2002. Centrosome amplification drives chromosomal instability in breast tumor development. *Proc. Natl. Acad. Sci. USA* **99:** 1978–1983.

49. Sotillo, R. *et al.* 2010. Mad2-induced chromosome instability leads to lung tumor relapse after oncogene withdrawal. *Nature* **464:** 436–440.

50. Teschendorff, A.E. & C. Caldas. 2009. The breast cancer somatic 'muta-ome': tackling the complexity. *Breast Cancer Res.* **11:** 301–305.

51. Wood, L.D. *et al.* 2007. The genomic landscapes of human breast and colorectal cancers. *Science* **318:** 1108–1113.

Ann. N.Y. Acad. Sci. ISSN 0077-8923

Predictive biomarkers in the management of EGFR mutant lung cancer

Rafael Rosell,[1,2] Teresa Moran,[1] Felipe Cardenal,[3] Rut Porta,[4] Santiago Viteri,[2] Miguel Angel Molina,[2] Susana Benlloch,[2] and Miquel Taron[1,2]

[1]Catalan Institue of Oncology, Hospital Germans Trias i Pujol, Badalona, Spain. [2]Pangaea Biotech, USP Dexeus University Institute, Barcelona, Spain. [3]Catalan Institute of Oncology, Hospital Duran Reynals, Bellvitge, Spain. [4]Catalan Institute of Oncology, Hospital Josep Trueta, Girona, Spain

Address for correspondence: Rafael Rosell, M.D., Catalan Institute of Oncology, Hospital Germans Trias i Pujol, Ctra Canyet, s/n, 08916 Badalona (Barcelona), Spain. rrosell@ico.scs.es

Activating mutations in the form of deletions in exon 19 (del 19) or the missense mutation L858R in the tyrosine kinase domain of the epidermal growth factor receptor (EGFR) predict outcome to use of EGFR tyrosine kinase inhibitors (TKIs), such as gefitinib and erlotinib. Pooled data from several phase II studies show that gefitinib and erlotinib induce responses in over 70% of NSCLC patients harboring EGFR mutations, with progression-free survival (PFS) ranging from 9 to 13 months. Two studies in Caucasian and Asian patients have confirmed that these subgroups of patients attain PFS up to 14 months. These landmark outcomes have been accompanied by new challenges, primarily the additional role of chemotherapy and the management of tumors with the secondary T790M mutation that confers resistance to EGFR TKIs. Mechanisms of resistance to reversible EGFR TKIs should be further clarified and could be related to modifications in DNA repair.

Keywords: non–small-cell lung cancer; EGFR mutations; serum DNA; gefitinib; erlotinib

Introduction

The concept underlying current cancer therapy is that patients with specific types and stages of cancer should be treated according to standardarized, predetermined protocols.[1] However, understanding the molecular genesis of cancer can lead to a rational use of targeted therapies. Imatinib, for example, is used for the treatment of major-breakpoint cluster region–Abelson murine leukemia viral oncogene homolog 1-positive (Bcr-Abl-positive) chronic myeloid leukemia (CML), and the reversible tyrosine kinase inhibitors (TKIs) erlotinib and gefitinib can block the mutated epidermal growth factor receptor (EGFR) protein expressed by some non-small cell lung cancers (NSCLC). Ninety percent of EGFR mutations are a deletion in exon 19 (del 19) or a missense mutation in exon 21 (L858R). These activating mutations stimulate three downstream signaling EGFR pathway components—PI3K, STAT, and RAS[2]—and eventually lead to the activation of five of the six hallmarks of cancer.[1]

A meta-analysis examined five small trials of first-line treatment with erlotinib or gefitinib monotherapy in patients in whom EGFR mutations were assessed.[3] In only one of the five trials were patients customized to receive gefitinib based on the presence of EGFR mutations.[4] A total of 317 chemotherapy-naive patients were treated with erlotinib or gefitinib, and tumor specimens from 223 of these patients were tested for EGFR mutations. Tumors from 84 patients were found to harbor EGFR mutations. Ninety percent of the EGFR-mutant patients were Caucasians.[3] The majority of EGFR-mutant patients were women (81%), had adenocarcinoma (89%), and had no history of tobacco use (58%). Of the 84 patients harboring a sensitizing EGFR mutation, treated with erlotinib or gefitinib, 56 patients (67%) achieved an objective response, with a median progression-free survival (PFS) of 11.8 months,

doi: 10.1111/j.1749-6632.2010.05775.x

and a median overall survival of 23.9 months. For 83 patients with wild-type EGFR and wild-type K-ras, the response rate was 5%, the median PFS was 3.1 months, and the median survival was 11.8 months. Finally, in 41 patients with wild-type EGFR and mutated K-ras, response was 0%, PFS 3.3 months, and median survival 13 months. As had been previously described,[5] patients with exon 19 deletions had a longer PFS (14.6 months vs. 9.7 months; $P = 0.02$) and overall survival (30.8 months vs. 14.8 months; $P < 0.001$) than those with the L858R mutation.[3] Outcomes of the 84 patients with EGFR mutations were also compared according to the EGFR TKI therapy; 56 patients received erlotinib and 28 received gefitinib. There were no significant differences in response rate (erlotinib 70%, gefitinib 60%; $P = 0.47$), median PFS (erlotinib 13 months, gefitinib 11.4 months; $P = 0.49$) or median survival (erlotinib 28.7 months, gefitinib 20.8 months; $P = 0.10$).[3]

In the meta-analysis,[3] patients were divided into two groups based on four major clinical predictors (race, gender, smoking status, and tumor histology): patients with three or four clinical predictors versus those with two or fewer. This clinical grouping helped to select a subset of clinically enriched patients with an increased likelihood of response (49% vs. 20%; $P < 0.001$) and prolonged median PFS (9.1 months vs. 4.4 months; $P = 0.01$). However, EGFR mutation status was a significantly better predictor of outcome. In the group of 59 patients with three or four clinical predictors (e.g., Asian, female, never-smoker, adenocarcinoma), EGFR mutation status was able to divide these patients into two clear subsets: 38 patients with sensitizing mutations (response 76%, PFS 12.9 months, and median survival 23.8 months) and 21 patients without a sensitizing mutation (response 0%, PFS 1.8 months, and median survival 14.8 months).

NSCLC cell lines with EGFR mutations

EGFR mutations were found in 13% of a large panel of non–small-cell lung carcinoma (NSCLC) cell lines; most of these mutant cell lines were derived from Caucasians, since 90% were established in the USA.[6] The frequency of EGFR mutations in these cell lines is similar to the 17% reported in clinical studies in Caucasian NSCLC patients.[7,8] Nine cell lines were sensitive to gefitinib, including seven of the ten mutated EGFR lines.[6] Interestingly, a re-

sponse rate of 70% has also been recently observed in patients with EGFR mutations treated with erlotinib[8] or gefitinib.[7]

The PC9 and H3255 cell lines had high sensitivity to EGFR TKIs. Interestingly, the EGFR signaling pathway positively regulates microRNA 21 (miR-21) expression. In the never-smoker-derived lung adenocarcinoma cell line H3255—with mutant EGFR and high levels of miR-21—antisense inhibition of miR-21 enhanced EGFR-TKI-induced apoptosis.[9] The H820 cell line—with intermediate sensitivity—was a mutated EGFR cell line having a secondary T790M mutation.[6] The resistant cell line category was the largest and included two mutated EGFR cell lines, one having the secondary T790M mutation (H1975) and the other (H1650) having homozygous deletion of the phosphatase and tensin homolog (PTEN) gene.[6] miR-21 can target and suppress PTEN,[10] but surprisingly, no increased miR-21 was observed in H1650 cells.[9] It is remarkable that the Scorpion Amplification Refractory Mutation system (SARMS) assay revealed that the frequency of the EGFR T790M was 55% for the H1975 but only 7% for the H820 cell line.[11] This poses the question of whether the amount of T790M could influence the length of PFS in NSCLC patients with EGFR mutations treated with EGFR TKIs (see below for further details).The remaining resistant cell lines in the Gandhi and colleagues study[6] included all of the wild-type EGFR cell lines and all lines having KRAS, BRAF, HER2, HER4, and PIK3CA mutations.[6] These findings mirror the clinical outcomes described above.[3]

The Spanish lung adenocarcinoma data base (SLADB)

The Spanish Lung Cancer Group evaluated the feasibility of large-scale screening of EGFR mutations in NSCLC patients and analyzed the association between EGFR mutations and clinical outcomes to erlotinib.[8] From April 2005 through November 2008, a total of 2,105 NSCLC patients from 129 institutions were prospectively screened for EGFR mutations. EGFR mutation assessment was performed centrally at the Catalan Institute of Oncology. The median time required for the EGFR mutation assay was 7 days from the time the sample arrived at the laboratory until the results were reported to the investigators. Mutations in the EGFR gene were detected in 350 of 2,105 patients (16.6%).

Table 1. Frequency of EGFR mutations

	All patients ($N = 2{,}105$)	Patients with EGFR mutations ($N = 350$)	Frequency among all 2,105 patients % (95% CI)	Frequency among 350 patients with mutations % (95% CI)
Gender*				
Female	814	244	30 (26.9–33.2)	69.71 (64.7–74.3)
Male	1,287	106	8.2 (6.8–9.9)	30.29 (25.7–35.3)
Age*				
≤56.7	638	89	13.9 (11.5–16.9)	27.05 (24.9–29.2)
56.7–69.1	638	99	15.5 (12.9–18.6)	30.1 (27.8–32.4)
>69.1	632	141	22.1 (19.1–25.6)	42.8 (40.2–45.5)
Smoking history*				
Ex-smoker	958	91	9.5 (7.8–11.6)	26.2 (24.2–28.2)
Current smoker	424	25	5.8 (4–8.6)	7.2 (6.5–7.9)
Never-smoker	612	231	37.7 (34–41.7)	66.6 (64.2–68.9)
Histology*				
Adeno	1,634	283	17.3 (15.5–19.3)	80.86 (76.4–84.7)
BAC	147	34	23.1 (17–30.7)	9.71 (7–13.3)
LCC	287	33	11.5 (8.3–15.8)	9.4 (6.8–13)

*Discrepancies in patient numbers are due to missing data.
Adeno, adenocarcinoma; BAC, bronchioloalveolar adenocarcinoma; LCC, large-cell carcinoma.

Mutations were detected more frequently in women (30%), never-smokers (37.7%), and adenocarcinomas (17.3%). However, mutations were also observed in men (8.2%), former smokers (9.5%) and even in current smokers (5.8%), and in large-cell carcinomas (11.5%)[8] (Table 1). Erlotinib was administered to 217 patients, of whom 113 received erlotinib as first-line therapy and 104 as second- or third-line therapy. EGFR del 19 mutations were detected in 135 tumors, and the L858R mutation in 82 tumors. Of the 164 patients in whom EGFR mutations were assessed also in serum, 97 carried mutations: del 19 in 64 patients and L858R in 33 patients. The overall response rate was 70.6%, including 12.2% complete responses[8] (Table 2). A better response was associated with the del 19 mutation than with the L858R mutation (odds ratio, 3.08; $P = 0.001$) and with an age between 61 and 70 years (odds ratio, 2.55; $P = 0.006$). Median PFS was 14 months (Fig. 1). The duration of response was similar for patients receiving first-line or second-line therapy. Median overall survival was 27 months. Median overall survival was 28 months for patients receiving first-line therapy and 27 months for those receiving second-line therapy.

Median PFS was 16 months in women and 9 months in men ($P = 0.003$). Median overall survival was 29 months in women and 18 months in men. There were no significant differences in progression-free survival according to performance status (PS), age, first-line versus second- or third-line therapy, or smoking history. The multivariate analysis revealed an association between poor PFS and male sex and the presence of the L858R mutation. In the multivariate analysis of overall survival, PS 1, male sex, the presence of the L858R mutation, brain metastases, and bronchioloalveolar adenocarcinoma were associated with poor prognosis.[8]

Clinical outcomes to gefitinib in Asian NSCLC patients with EGFR mutations have recently been reviewed.[12]

Development of acquired drug resistance by mutation of the gatekeeper T790 residue

The clinical efficacy of gefitinib or erlotinib is limited by the development of acquired drug resistance that is believed to be caused by the T790M mutation, which is detected in 50% of clinically resistant patients.[13,14] Serial analyses of EGFR-mutated patients treated with gefitinib or erlotinib revealed the

Table 2. Patient characteristics and response for 217 patients receiving erlotinib

	N (%)
Age, median (range)	67 (22–88)
Gender	
Male	59 (27.2)
Female	158 (72.8)
Race	
African	3 (1.4)
Asian	1 (0.5)
Caucasian	213 (98.2)
Smoking history	
Ex-smoker	56 (25.8)
Current smoker	13 (6)
Never-smoker	148 (68.2)
ECOG PS	
0	51 (23.5)
1	128 (58.9)
≥2	38 (17.6)
Histology	
Adeno	176 (81.1)
BAC	22 (10.1)
LCC	19 (8.8)
Stage	
IIIB	12 (5.5)
IV	205 (94.5)
Erlotinib treatment line	
First	113 (52.1)
Second	104 (47.9)
EGFR mutation	
del 19	135 (62.2)
L858R	82 (37.8)
EGFR mutation in serum ($N = 164$)	
del 19	64 (39)
L858R	33 (20)
not detected	67 (41)
Response	
CR	24 (12.2)
PR	115 (58.4)
CR + PR	139 (70.6)
	(95% CI : 63.8–76.5)
SD	38 (19.3)
PD	20 (10.2)
SD + PD	58 (29.4)
NE	20

Adeno, adenocarcinoma; BAC, bronchioloalveolar adenocarcinoma; LCC, large-cell carcinoma.

increased prevalence of the resistant T790M mutation in circulating tumor cells over time.[15] The T790M mutation has also been detected in pretreatment specimens.[16] SARMS identified the T790M mutation in pretreatment tumor samples from 10 of 26 patients (38%). The T790M mutation was associated with a strikingly short PFS—a median of 7.7 months in patients with the T790M mutation and 16.5 months in those without the mutation (hazard ratio for progression for the T790M allele, 11.5; $P < 0.001$).[15] Scorpion amplification refractory mutation system (SARMS) in combination with another method identified T790M in 70% of post-treatment biopsy specimens and in plasma DNA in 54% of patients with prior response to gefitinib or erlotinib and in 29% of patients with prior stable disease.[11]

The expression levels of DNA repair genes involved in homologous recombination and non-homologous end joining could influence PFS to erlotinib. Figure 2 illustrates the prognostic role of breast cancer 1 (BRCA1) mRNA levels in patients with EGFR mutations, including those with double mutations. This could serve as a model for future treatment approaches, as shown in Figure 2.

The centrality of the BRCA1 pathway in DNA damage response to different types of genotoxic stress

A large-scale proteomic analysis of proteins phosphorylated in response to DNA damage on consensus sites recognized by ataxia telangiectasia mutated (ATM) and ataxia telangiectasia and Rad3 related (ATR) identified more than 900 regulated phosphorylation sites, encompassing over 700 proteins.[17] This set of proteins is highly interconnected, with a large number of protein modules and networks not previously linked to DNA damage response.[17] In our opinion, a module that is central to DNA damage response is BRCA1, which includes BRCA1-associated ring domain protein (BARD1), BRCA2, partner and localizer of BRCA2 (PALPB2), ATM, and E2F transcription factor 1 (E2F1). This module also contains RAD51 homolog (RAD51) and X-ray repair complementing defective repair in Chinese hamster cells 3 (XRCC3) (which are related to homologous recombination repair) and replication protein A (RPA) and excision repair cross-complementing rodent repair deficiency, complementation group 1 (ERCC1).

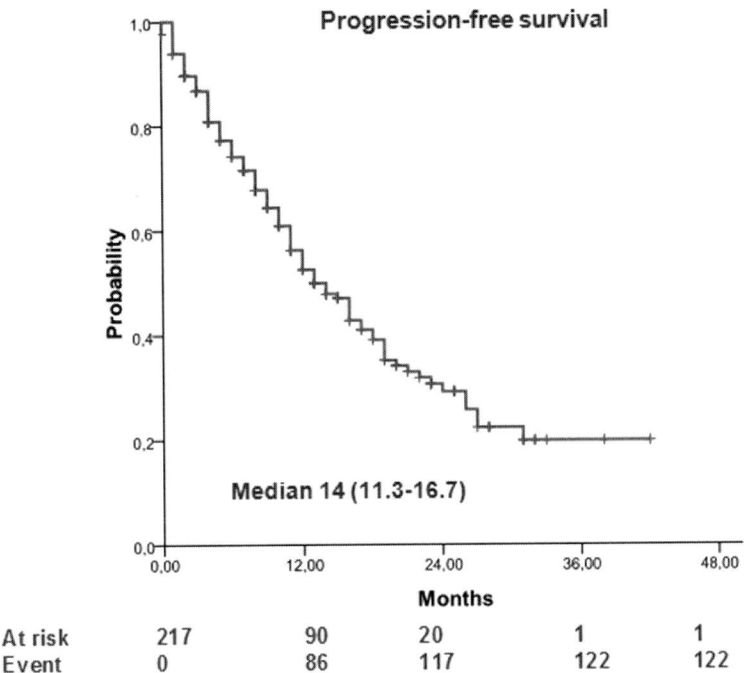

Figure 1. Progression-free survival in NSCLC patients with EGFR mutations treated with erlotinib.[8]

In stage IIIA NSCLC patients treated with neoadjuvant cisplatin/gemcitabine, median survival was not reached in those with low BRCA1 mRNA levels, while those with high BRCA1 mRNA levels had a median survival of one year and no long-term survival.[18] These results prompted us to examine whether customizing treatment by BRCA1 levels could improve outcome in advanced NSCLC patients.

From 2005 to 2007, we performed a non-randomized phase II trial of customized treatment based on EGFR mutation status and BRCA1 mRNA expression levels. We opted to limit enrollment to non-squamous cell carcinoma in order to maximize the opportunity to administer erlotinib in patients with EGFR mutations. Patients with either the exon 19 deletion or the L858R mutation received erlotinib, while those with wild-type EGFR received chemotherapy based on BRCA1 levels: those with low levels received cisplatin plus gemcitabine; those with intermediate levels received cisplatin plus docetaxel; and those with high levels received docetaxel alone. Median survival exceeded 28 months for 12 patients with EGFR mutations, and was 11 months for 38 patients with low BRCA1, 9 months for 40 patients with intermediate BRCA1, and 11 months

for 33 patients with high BRCA1. Two-year survival was 73.3%, 41.2%, 15.6%, and 0%, respectively.

Genotoxic stress, including chemotherapy response, is related to the fact that DNA repair genes require a series of molecular recognition steps that enable DNA damage response proteins to localize at and near DNA lesions. Binding of the mediator of DNA damage checkpoint 1 protein to the phosphorylated tail of histone H2AX (γH2AX) facilitates the formation of BRCA1 nuclear foci at double-strand breaks induced by irradiation or chemotherapy. By dimerizing with BARD1 protein through the RING domain, BRCA1 forms an E3 ubiquitin ligase.

Sensitivity of different EGFR mutation assays

In the earlier studies, direct sequencing was commonly used for the detection of EGFR mutations.[19–22] However, as direct sequencing can only detect mutant sequences constituting >30% of the total genetic content, it is not generally useful for the detection of EGFR mutations in body fluids in which only a small fraction of the EGFR sequences are mutants. Nevertheless, because of the clinical importance of identifying EGFR mutations in NSCLC for customized therapy,[7,8] cytological samples should

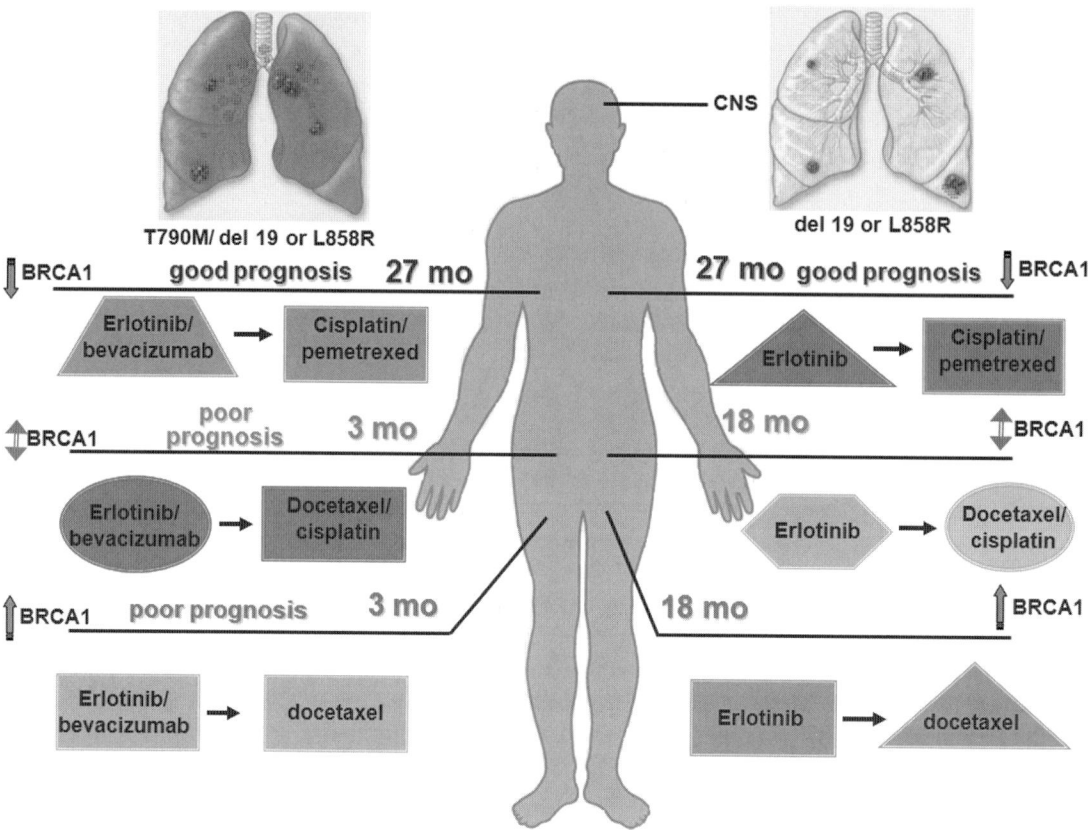

Figure 2. A hypothetical model based on the experience of the SLADB study, where patients with low BRCA1 mRNA expression attained PFS of up to 27 months, which declined as BRCA1 expression increased. Erlotinib can cause double-strand breaks that are repaired by homologous recombination. The figure also illustrates the potential use of different EGFR TKIs based on the presence of double mutations and customized chemotherapy options at the time of failure to erlotinib.

not be dismissed as inadequate without a thorough review. At present, any cytology cell block specimen with at least 25% of tumor cells should be deemed adequate for EGFR mutational analysis by direct sequencing[23]. In general, pleural fluids have the most material of all cytologic samples. The absolute amount of cancer on the sections is less critical than the homogeneity of the sections, and by dissecting ten 5-μm sections, adequate DNA could be obtained from regions of cancer as small as 2 mm² and with as few as 40 cancer cells[23]. Molina-Vila and colleagues[24] have developed a method that permits detection of del 19, L858R, and T790M in samples containing as few as eight tumor cells (in 10 μl of buffer), approximately 5pg of DNA per microliter of crude extract. This method is based on microdissecting tumor cells directly into polymerase chain reaction (PCR) buffer, followed by amplification and determination of EGFR status by length

analysis of fluorescently-labeled products (del 19) or TaqMan assay (L858R and T790M).[24] In addition to direct sequencing, EGFR mutations can be assessed by common fragment analysis of PCR-mediated amplification products (del 19), by real-time PCR (L858R), or by the peptide nucleic acid-locked nucleic acid PCR clamp method.[8,24,25] SARMS has also been used,[7,11,26] as has the DxS EGFR29 mutation-detection kit.[7]

Monoclonal antibodies against del 19 and L858R have shown a sensitivity of 92% by immunohistochemistry.[27] Pathologists have observed that EGFR mutations are particularly frequent in the papillary and acinar subtypes of adenocarcinoma,[28] and that those patients with adenocarcinomas with a solid pattern harboring EGFR mutations had a shorter PFS to erlotinib.[28] We have also observed a shorter PFS (10 months) to erlotinib in solid adenocarcinomas.[8] Interestingly 73% of micropapillary adenocarcinomas harbored mutually exclusive mutations: K-ras (33%), EGFR (20%), and BRAF (20%).[29]

EGFR mutations in circulating plasma or serum DNA

The assessment of EGFR mutations in circulating DNA involves several important facets. The monitoring of EGFR mutations in blood can quantify the level of EGFR mutations with highly sensitive digital PCR assays, making it a useful method to define a molecular response and to identify disease progression. A discordance of 27% in the presence of EGFR mutations between primary tumors and metastases has been reported; in some cases, the mutations were present in the primary tumor but not in the metastasis, while in other cases, the opposite phenomenon occurred.[30] In addition, in a few instances, EGFR mutations have been observed in plasma DNA but not in the tumor.[11] Using SARMS, EGFR mutations were identified in 33% of cases in plasma but in 92% of cases in circulating tumor cells.[15] We identified EGFR mutations in circulating DNA in 97 of 164 patients with available paired tumor-serum samples using the peptide nucleic acid-locked nucleic acid PCR clamp method.[8] The frequency in serum increased up to 75% in patients with more than one metastatic site and to 80% in patients with poor PS.[8] Denaturing high-performance liquid chromatography (DHPLC) has also been used to analyze EGFR mutations in paired tumor-plasma samples,[31] with a high degree of concordance. Importantly, the correlation between treatment response and plasma concentration of mutated EGFR sequences might be useful for the detection of clinical relapse[32] as well as to define complete molecular remission—a term that is not often used in NSCLC with EGFR mutations but is common in chronic myeloid leukemia (CML). In microfluidics digital PCR analysis, template DNA molecules are distributed into multiple reaction vessels so that the average number of DNA molecules in each reaction vessel is <1.[32] Digital PCR assays were able to detect a mutant molecule in a background of wild-type sequences at a fractional concentration of 0.1%. Interestingly, the quantification of mutant sequences by digital PCR analysis is performed through the physical counting of the number of positive reactions and hence does not require calibration standards for generating calibration curves.[32] In addition to sensitively detecting the circulating EGFR mutations, the digital PCR assays are able to measure the concentrations of the mutant sequences.

Conclusions

NSCLC-specific EGFR mutations are the first target for selective treatment identified in NSCLC, with an importance similar to that of Bcr-Abl in CML. Clinical outcomes in our prospective study of customized erlotinb[8] represent a new landmark in lung cancer management: 70% overall response rate (including 12% complete responses), a median PFS of 14 months (even longer in women and in patients with del 19), 20% of patients without disease progression at three years, and a median survival of 27 months. These are unprecedented findings in the treatment of lung cancer. Nonetheless, these clinical outcomes fall short of curability, and continuous treatment with erlotinib or gefitinib is required. It is plausible that several genetically defined subclasses of EGFR mutations could help to improve current clinical outcomes by combining erlotinib or gefitinib with other targeted drugs.

Conflicts of Interest

The authors declare no conflicts of interest.

References

1. Gazdar, A.F. 2009. Personalized medicine and inhibition of EGFR signaling in lung cancer. *N. Engl. J. Med.* **361:** 1018–1020.
2. Sordella, R. *et al.* 2004. Gefitinib-sensitizing EGFR mutations in lung cancer activate anti-apoptotic pathways. *Science* **305:** 1163–1167.
3. Jackman, D.M. *et al.* 2009. Impact of epidermal growth factor receptor and KRAS mutations on clinical outcomes in previously untreated non-small cell lung cancer patients: results of an online tumor registry of clinical trials. *Clin. Cancer Res.* **15:** 5267–5273.
4. Sequist, L.V. *et al.* 2008. First-line gefitinib in patients with advanced non-small-cell lung cancer harboring somatic EGFR mutations. *J. Clin. Oncol.* **26:** 2442–2449.
5. Riely, G.J. *et al.* 2006. Clinical course of patients with non-small cell lung cancer and epidermal growth factor receptor exon 19 and exon 21 mutations treated with gefitinib or erlotinib. *Clin. Cancer Res.* **12:** 839–844.
6. Gandhi, J. *et al.* 2009. Alterations in genes of the EGFR signaling pathway and their relationship to EGFR tyrosine kinase inhibitor sensitivity in lung cancer cell lines. *PLoS ONE* **4:** e4576.
7. Mok, T.S. *et al.* 2009. Gefitinib or carboplatin-paclitaxel in pulmonary adenocarcinoma. *N. Engl. J. Med.* **361:** 947–957.

8. Rosell, R. *et al.* 2009. Screening for epidermal growth factor receptor mutations in lung cancer. *N. Engl. J. Med.* **361:** 958–967.

9. Seike, M. *et al.* 2009. MiR-21 is an EGFR-regulated anti-apoptotic factor in lung cancer in never-smokers. *Proc. Natl. Acad. Sci. USA* **106:** 12085–12090.

10. Meng, F. *et al.* 2007. MicroRNA-21 regulates expression of the PTEN tumor suppressor gene in human hepatocellular cancer. *Gastroenterology* **133:** 647–658.

11. Kuang, Y. *et al.* 2009. Noninvasive detection of EGFR T790M in gefitinib or erlotinib resistant non-small cell lung cancer. *Clin. Cancer Res.* **15:** 2630–2636.

12. Rosell, R. *et al.* 2009. Epidermal growth factor receptor tyrosine kinase inhibitors as first-line treatment in advanced nonsmall-cell lung cancer. *Curr. Opin. Oncol.* **22:** 112–120.

13. Nguyen, K.S., S. Kobayashi & D.B. Costa. 2009. Acquired resistance to epidermal growth factor receptor tyrosine kinase inhibitors in non-small-cell lung cancers dependent on the epidermal growth factor receptor pathway. *Clin. Lung Cancer* **10:** 281–289.

14. Zhou, W. *et al.* 2009. Novel mutant-selective EGFR kinase inhibitors against EGFR T790M. *Nature* **462:** 1070–1074.

15. Maheswaran, S. *et al.* 2008. Detection of mutations in EGFR in circulating lung-cancer cells. *N. Engl. J. Med.* **359:** 366–377.

16. Inukai, M. *et al.* 2006. Presence of epidermal growth factor receptor gene T790M mutation as a minor clone in non-small cell lung cancer. *Cancer Res.* **66:** 7854–7858.

17. Matsuoka, S. *et al.* 2007. ATM and ATR substrate analysis reveals extensive protein networks responsive to DNA damage. *Science* **316:** 1160–1166.

18. Taron, M. *et al.* 2004. BRCA1 mRNA expression levels as an indicator of chemoresistance in lung cancer. *Hum. Mol. Genet.* **13:** 2443–2449.

19. Lynch, T.J. *et al.* 2004. Activating mutations in the epidermal growth factor receptor underlying responsiveness of non-small-cell lung cancer to gefitinib. *N. Engl. J. Med.* **350:** 2129–2139.

20. Paez, J.G. *et al.* 2004. EGFR mutations in lung cancer: correlation with clinical response to gefitinib therapy. *Science* **304:** 1497–1500.

21. Pao, W. *et al.* 2004. EGF receptor gene mutations are common in lung cancers from "never smokers" and are associated with sensitivity of tumors to gefitinib and erlotinib. *Proc. Natl. Acad. Sci. USA* **101:** 13306–13311.

22. Taron, M. *et al.* 2005. Activating mutations in the tyrosine kinase domain of the epidermal growth factor receptor are associated with improved survival in gefitinib-treated chemorefractory lung adenocarcinomas. *Clin. Cancer Res.* **11:** 5878–5885.

23. Smouse, J.H. *et al.* 2009. EGFR mutations are detected comparably in cytologic and surgical pathology specimens of nonsmall cell lung cancer. *Cancer Cytopathol.* **117:** 67–72.

24. Molina-Vila, M.A. *et al.* 2008. A sensitive method for detecting EGFR mutations in non-small cell lung cancer samples with few tumor cells. *J. Thorac. Oncol.* **3:** 1224–1235.

25. Morita, S. *et al.* 2009. Combined survival analysis of prospective clinical trials of gefitinib for non-small cell lung cancer with EGFR mutations. *Clin. Cancer Res.* **15:** 4493–4498.

26. Miyazawa, H. *et al.* 2008. Peptide nucleic acid-locked nucleic acid polymerase chain reaction clamp-based detection test for gefitinib-refractory T790M epidermal growth factor receptor mutation. *Cancer Sci.* **99:** 595–600.

27. Yu, J. *et al.* 2009. Mutation-specific antibodies for the detection of EGFR mutations in non-small-cell lung cancer. *Clin. Cancer Res.* **15:** 3023–3028.

28. Motoi, N. *et al.* 2008. Lung adenocarcinoma: modification of the 2004 WHO mixed subtype to include the major histologic subtype suggests correlations between papillary and micropapillary adenocarcinoma subtypes, EGFR mutations and gene expression analysis. *Am. J. Surg. Pathol.* **32:** 810–827.

29. De Oliveira Duarte Achcar, R., M.N. Nikiforova & S.A. Yousem. 2009. Micropapillary lung adenocarcinoma: EGFR, K-ras, and BRAF mutational profile. *Am. J. Clin. Pathol.* **131:** 694–700.

30. Gow, C.H. *et al.* 2009. Comparison of epidermal growth factor receptor mutations between primary and corresponding metastatic tumors in tyrosine kinase inhibitor-naive non-small-cell lung cancer. *Ann. Oncol.* **20:** 696–702.

31. Bai, H. *et al.* 2009. Epidermal growth factor receptor mutations in plasma DNA samples predict tumor response in Chinese patients with stages IIIB to IV non-small-cell lung cancer. *J. Clin. Oncol.* **27:** 2653–2659.

32. Yung, T.K. *et al.* 2009. Single-molecule detection of epidermal growth factor receptor mutations in plasma by microfluidics digital PCR in non-small cell lung cancer patients. *Clin. Cancer Res.* **15:** 2076–2084.

Ann. N.Y. Acad. Sci. ISSN 0077-8923

ANNALS OF THE NEW YORK ACADEMY OF SCIENCES

Issue: *Toward Personalized Medicine for Cancer*

Primary trastuzumab resistance: new tricks for an old drug

Jason A. Wilken[1] and Nita J. Maihle[1,2]

[1]Yale University, School of Medicine, Department of Obstetrics, Gynecology, and Reproductive Sciences, New Haven, Connecticut. [2]Yale University, School of Medicine, Departments of Pathology and Pharmacology, New Haven, Connecticut

Address for correspondence: Nita J. Maihle, Ph.D., P.O. Box 208063, 310 Cedar St., New Haven, CT 06520-8063. nita.maihle@yale.edu

Trastuzumab is the first Food and Drug Administration (FDA)-approved therapeutic targeting a HER-family receptor tyrosine kinase (HER2/ErbB2/neu). Although trastuzumab is effective in the treatment of HER2-positive breast cancer, a substantial proportion of patients will not respond to trastuzumab-based regimens (primary resistance), and those who do respond will often lose clinical benefits (i.e., secondary resistance). Although multiple mechanisms underlying the development of secondary trastuzumab resistance have been identified, few studies have specifically examined the basis of primary trastuzumab resistance. Here, we review these studies, which together demonstrate that trastuzumab induces phenotypic changes in tumor cells, even when they are not growth inhibited by trastuzumab, including changes in gene expression. These changes have important clinical implications, including the sensitization of malignant cells to other therapeutic drugs. In light of these observations, we propose that the conventional definition of *resistance* as it pertains to trastuzumab and, perhaps, to other targeted therapeutics, may require revision. The results of these studies will be useful in informing the direction of future basic and clinical research focused on overcoming primary trastuzumab resistance.

Keywords: EGFR/ErbB/HER; trastuzumab/herceptin; breast cancer; targeted therapeutics; primary resistance

Introduction

Although the HER2-directed antibody trastuzumab is one of the early success stories among biologically targeted breast cancer therapeutics, some patients will not respond to this drug, and among responders, the majority will eventually relapse. This clinical scenario occurs in spite of steadfast efforts to select patients for trastuzumab treatment on the basis of HER2-positive tumor status with expensive diagnostic tests.[1] Here, we review recent studies on the mechanistic basis of primary trastuzumab resistance. These studies suggest that multiple endpoints beyond tumor cell growth inhibition should be considered during the evaluation of trastuzumab efficacy, and perhaps the efficacy of other emerging biologically targeted therapeutics.

Proposed mechanisms of trastuzumab activity

Contrary to initial assumptions, trastuzumab does not appear to inhibit HER2 dimerization or ligand-dependent HER heterodimeric signaling.[2] Instead, three major mechanisms of trastuzumab inhibition of tumor growth and survival have gained some experimental support:

(1) targeting of immune cells to HER2-positive tumor cells: Immune cells, binding to trastuzumab Fc domains, affect antibody-dependent cell-mediated cytotoxicity (ADCC) of HER2-positive tumor cells.[3–5]

(2) inhibition of HER2 shedding: In certain breast cancer-derived cell lines, the extracellular domain (ECD) of HER2 is proteolytically shed from the cell surface,[6–8] and the remaining truncated receptor ("p95HER2" or "t95HER2",[9]), now freed from autoinhibition by the receptor's ECD, exhibits constitutive tyrosine kinase activity.[10,11] Trastuzumab binding to the HER2 receptor inhibits proteolytic shedding, perhaps via a steric or allosteric mechanism, resulting in decreased HER2 kinase activity.[10] This model is discussed in the

doi: 10.1111/j.1749-6632.2010.05782.x

context of recent studies demonstrating that p95HER2 also may be expressed from an alternate HER2 transcript (see section IV).[12]

(3) internalization and degradation of HER2: Trastuzumab binding to HER2 stimulates the recruitment of c-Cbl and resulting in subsequent HER2 ubiquitinlyation, internalization, and degradation.[13–15]

Given the diversity of these proposed mechanisms of trastuzumab's therapeutic activity, it is perhaps not surprizing that our understanding of trastuzumab resistance, both primary and secondary, is incomplete. Although the mechanistic basis for secondary resistance recently has been reviewed,[16–18] the number of studies exploring the mechanistic basis of primary trastuzumab resistance is relatively limited. Here, we review several recent studies on the mechanism of primary resistance to trastuzumab, and discuss unifying themes revealed by them.

Clinical studies reveal complex patterns of responsiveness to trastuzumab

Most patients with early stage breast cancer, and a large proportion of patients with metastatic breast cancer, have a measurable tumor response to trastuzumab chemotherapy, as demonstrated by a reduction in tumor burden (i.e., partial or complete response). However, a fraction (∼20%) of early stage breast cancer patients will not respond to trastuzumab, and ∼70% of patients with metastatic disease who receive trastuzumab monotherapy are resistant to treatment.[19,20] De novo or "primary" resistance occurs when trastuzumab is ineffective for the treatment of breast cancer patients, despite tumor expression of HER2. "Acquired" or "secondary" trastuzumab resistance occurs when patients who initially respond to trastuzumab experience trastuzumab-refractory relapse. Patients with HER2-positive breast cancer are typically treated with a combination of trastuzumab and chemotherapy, as exemplified in the pivotal National Surgical Adjuvant Breast and Bowel Project B31 and NC-CTG N9831 trials. In both of these studies, although the addition of trastuzumab to chemotherapy reduced the chance of death among patients with early-stage HER2-positive breast cancer, survival among patients treated with chemotherapy alone was also high.[21] Because patients are not routinely

treated with trastuzumab monotherapy, the relative contribution of each drug to reduced tumor burden, as well as the potential interactions among these drugs, can be difficult to assess, and both primary and secondary trastuzumab resistance must necessarily be associated with primary resistance to genotoxic therapies as well as to trastuzumab (except in the case of neoadjuvant trastuzumab monotherapy).

Putative mechanisms of primary trastuzumab resistance

Most studies on trastuzumab resistance have focused on the mechanisms underlying acquired or secondary trastuzumab resistance, using trastuzumab-sensitive cell lines such as SKBR3 and BT474 cultured with trastuzumab until a resistant phenotype emerges. Several recent studies, however, have examined in vitro models of primary trastuzumab resistance, or have studied the properties of trastuzumab-resistant tumors, to explore the mechanistic basis for this phenomenon. The results of these studies are summarized schematically in Figure 1, and are discussed in more detail below.

N-terminal truncation of HER2
Alternate isoforms of all four members of the HER family have been described.[9] Soluble (s) HER2 isoforms arise from alternately spliced transcripts of the HER2 gene resulting in 68 kDa[22] or 100 kDa[23] isoforms encompassing most of the HER2 ECD, or from proteolytic cleavage of full-length HER2 resulting in shed 105 kDa[7] or 110 kDa[6,8] sHER2 fragments of the ECD. Proteolytic cleavage of full-length HER2 also yields a cell-surface associated fragment of ∼95 kDa (termed "p95HER2") encompassing a small fragment of the ECD, the transmembrane domain, and the intracellular domain (including the tyrosine kinase).[11]

Although all of these isoforms may be relevant to clinical targeting of HER2 in cancer patients, it is the p95HER2 product that has received the most attention to date. Specifically, p95HER2, freed from ECD-mediated autoinhibition, is a constitutively active kinase and a potent oncogene.[24] Since p95HER2 lacks the trastuzumab-binding domain of full-length HER2 (see Fig. 1, panel B), it may also be an important mediator of primary trastuzumab resistance. Preclinical xenograft studies demonstrate that T47D[12] and MCF7[25] cells stably

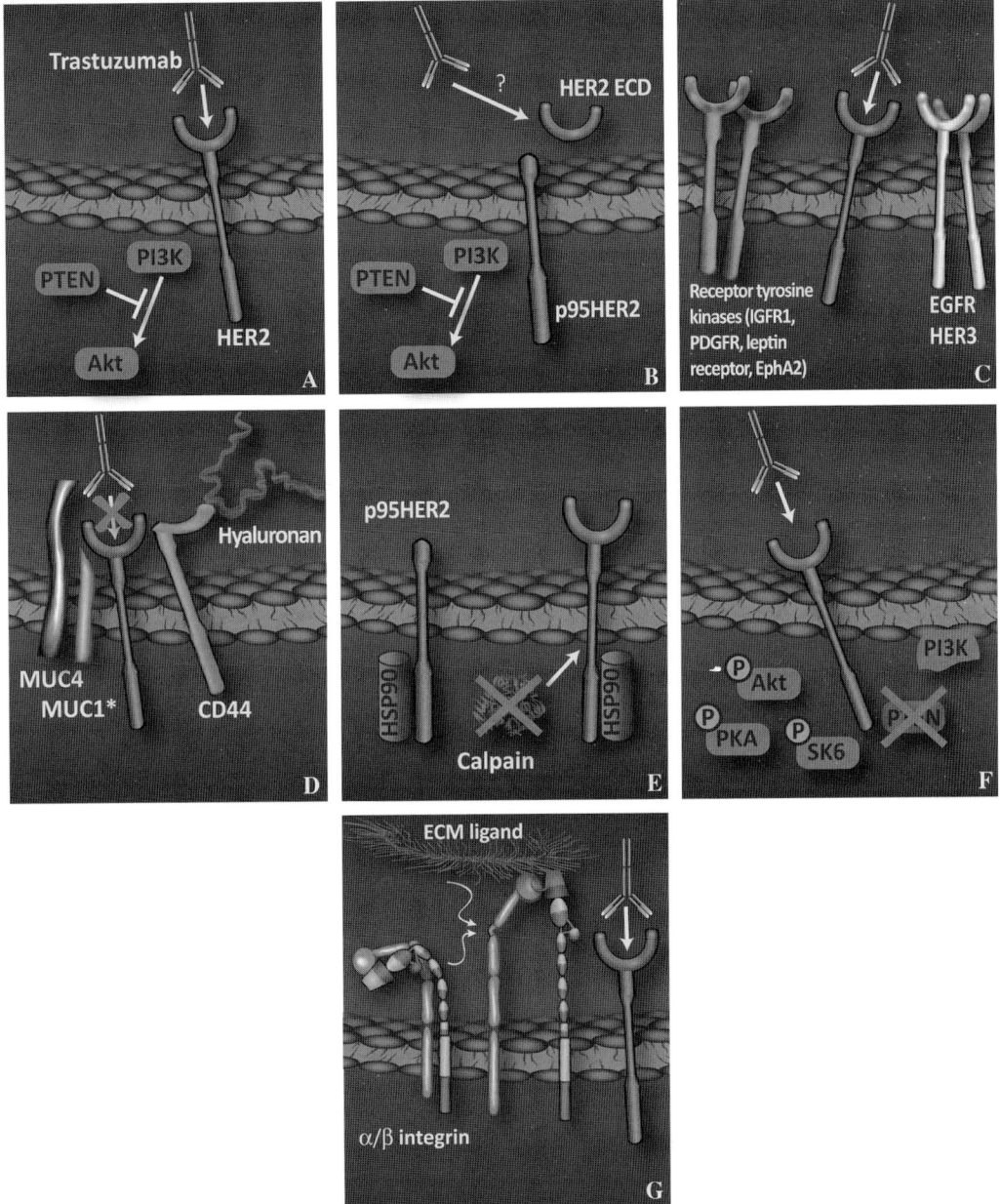

Figure 1. Potential mechanisms underlying primary trastuzumab resistance. (A) Although the proposed mechanisms of trastuzumab action are diverse (and are not mutually exclusive), one consensus viewpoint is that trastuzumab must be able to bind to the HER2 extracellular domain, and in doing so this antibody inhibits the association of PI3K and activated HER2, which leads to decreased activation of Akt and subsequent inhibition of cell proliferation and survival. Even in the absence of a unifying hypothesis for the mechanism of trastuzumab inhibition of tumor cell growth, several alternate mechanisms to define the basis for primary trastuzumab resistance have been reported as summarized in this review, and are depicted schematically here. (B) Expression or proteolytic generation of p95HER2, a constitutively kinase-active HER2 isoform lacking the trastuzumab-binding site. (C) Compensatory signaling by other cell surface receptors, including EGFR/HER3 and other receptor tyrosine kinases. (D) Physical blockade of trastuzumab/HER2 association by CD44/hyaluronin, MUC1*, or MUC4. (E) Increased HER2 stability in association with chaperone/HER2 interaction or downregulation of HER2-client proteases. (F) Constitutive activation of downstream effectors or crosstalk pathways. (G) Interaction of integrins and extracellular matrix components, resulting in enhanced HER2-independent cell proliferation survival signaling. (H) Dispensability of HER2 (not displayed). In this model, HER2 expression may be stochastic and nonessential in some tumor cells.

expressing p95HER2 are insensitive to trastuzumab, whereas cells stably expressing full-length HER2 are growth inhibited by trastuzumab. Although retrospective studies have associated p95HER2 expression with an aggressive breast tumor phenotype and poor patient outcome,[26,27] only two studies have specifically examined the role of p95HER2 in primary trastuzumab resistance in breast cancer. Scaltriti and colleagues[25] and Sperinde and colleagues[28] both demonstrate an association between p95HER2 expression and failure to respond to primary trastuzumab regimens

Regulation of p95HER2 expression reveals additional complexities of the primary trastuzumab-resistant phenotype. Initial studies demonstrated that full-length HER2 can be cleaved by a metalloprotease resulting in the generation of a p95HER2 membrane-associated fragment and a "shed" ECD fragment[6–8]; moreover, trastuzumab inhibits HER2 ECD shedding.[10] However, recent studies have identified an alternate transcript of HER2 that encodes a p95HER2 isoform lacking most or all of the ECD.[12] The relative contribution of these two distinct mechanisms to the synthesis of p95HER2 in tumor cells has not been determined, nor has the potential role of the shed ECD (or alternate sHER2 isoform[s]) been examined in the context of primary trastuzumab resistance.

Might the proteolytically shed sHER2 (ECD) isoform also play a role in primary trastuzumab resistance? Early studies by Brodowicz and colleagues[29] demonstrated that sHER2 ECD, perhaps acting as an antibody sink, attenuated growth inhibitory effects of anti-HER2 antibodies on HER2-positive breast cancer cell lines (see Fig. 1, panel B). More recent studies by Ghedini and colleagues[30] suggest that sHER2 may serve to bind to and deliver trastuzumab to the cell surface thereby synergistically inhibiting the growth of HER2-positive cells. Clinical correlative studies on circulating sHER2 have demonstrated a trend—or statistically significant correlation—between decline in posttreatment versus baseline serum sHER2 concentration and responsiveness to trastuzumab therapy.[31–33] However, the limited biochemical characterization of this circulating isoform(s) of sHER2, as well as the limited number of functional studies on serum sHER2, prevent us from concluding that this isoform plays an active role in the development of primary trastuzumab resistance.

Dispensability and redundancy of HER2 signaling

Arnould and colleagues[34] demonstrated that primary trastuzumab resistance was inversely associated with breast cancer HER2 expression. Complementary studies by Ginester and colleagues have identified basal phosphorylation of HER2 as a predictor of trastuzumab resistance in vitro; in these studies primary trastuzumab resistance was common among basal-subtype cell lines and/or cell lines with low basal levels of phosphorylation of HER2.[35] Although the mechanism underlying reduced basal HER2 phosphorylation was not rigorously characterized in this study, the lack of constitutive HER2 phosphorylation in these cells suggests that HER2 may not an "addictive oncogene" under these conditions, in contrast to its role in BT-474 and SKBR-3 cells.[36]

Complementary evidence in support of the dispensability or redundancy of HER2 signaling in certain breast carcinoma-derived cell lines has been reported by Narayan and colleagues[37] In this study, several cell lines were selected that were not growth inhibited by trastuzumab or by epidermal growth factor receptor (EGFR/ErbB1/HER1) inhibitors; long-term trastuzumab treatment sensitized these cells to EGFR inhibitor-mediated growth inhibition suggesting that HER2 and EGFR signaling may be compensatory in these cell lines, i.e., only one functional HER axis is required for cell proliferation. This concept is further supported by recent observations showing that trastuzumab-mediated growth inhibition can be overcome by ectopic expression of EGFR in SKBR3 cells[38] or HB-EGF treatment of BT474 cells.[39] Similarly, an inhibitor of heparin binding epidermal growth factor (HB-EGF) renders MCF7–HER2 cells sensitive to trastuzumab.[39] High tumor EGFR expression levels also have been associated with primary resistance to trastuzumab neoadjuvant therapy.[40]

Similarly, in two studies, mRNA profiles of pretreatment breast tumor core biopsies were compared in patients with complete versus noncomplete pathologic response to trastuzumab in a neoadjuvant setting. Harris and colleagues demonstrated that unresponsive patients (trastuzumab plus vinorelbine) were found to have elevated tumor expression levels of wnt family members, growth factors, and growth factor receptors such as HGF, met, IGF-I, PDGF, leptin receptor, and pleitoropin; increased expression of IGF-1 in primary trastuzumab-resistant breast tumors was confirmed by immunohistochemistry (see Fig. 1, Panel C).[19] More recent studies have demonstrated that IGFBP3, an inhibitor of IGF-1, synergizes with trastuzumab to inhibit the growth of primary trastuzumab-resistant cells.[41,42] By contrast, Vegran and colleagues[43] did not identify growth factor receptors as part of a gene array profile upregulated in nonresponsive (trastuzumab plus docetaxel) patient tumors, but did identify upregulation of certain cell signaling effectors in tumor samples from nonresponsive patients (see below).

In vitro studies also have identified the receptor tyrosine kinase EphA2 as commonly overexpressed in breast cancer cell lines resistant to trastuzumab, but not in cell lines sensitive to trastuzumab,[44] and EphA2 expression also has been correlated with poor survival in breast cancer patients.[45,46] However, not all cell surface receptors cooperate to attenuate trastuzumab sensitivity. For example, granulocyte-colony stimulating factor in combination with trastuzumab can synergistically induce apoptosis in the primary trastuzumab-resistant cell lines T47D and ZR-75-1.[47] These studies illustrate the complex effect of cytokines on trastuzumab's activity in tumor cells, and also the importance of considering the entire complement of tyrosine kinases in the context of the tumor cell's resistance to trastuzumab.

Steric access to receptor and HER2 stability

As outlined above, several competing hypotheses have been proposed for the mechanism(s) of trastuzumab-mediated inhibition of tumor cell growth (see "Proposed mechanisms of trastuzumab activity", above). One unifying aspect among these mechanisms is that tumor cell growth inhibition is dependent on the binding of trastuzumab to the ECD of HER2. Therefore, processes or molecules that mask or prevent trastuzumab from binding to the HER2 receptor would be predicted to block trastuzumab activity. Experimental support for this hypothesis is summarized below.

Associations between HER2 and other cell surface signaling proteins, i.e., integrin β1,[48] and CD44 (hyaluronin receptor),[49] have been associated with primary trastuzumab resistance in the breast cancer-derived cell line JIMT-1 (see Fig. 1, panel D). Studies using this cell line suggest that reduced trastuzumab

binding to cell surface HER2 is mediated by steric hindrance associated with CD44 and/or MUC4 expression. This concept is supported by the observation that 4-methylumbelliferon, a hyaluronin synthesis inhibitor, increases trastuzumab binding to JIMT-1 cells, resulting in synergistic inhibition of JIMT-1 xenograft growth.[49] Similarly, MUC4, a high-molecular mass proteoglycan, coimmunoprecipitates with HER2 from lysates of JIMT-1 cells, and also inhibits cell surface binding of trastuzumab.[50] In further support of this concept, siRNA's directed against MUC4 increase trastuzumab binding to JIMT-1 cells.[51] Clearly, however, HER2 association with CD44 and/or MUC4 does not completely inhibit trastuzumab binding to JIMT-1 cells, nor does this association mask all HER2 epitopes, because pertuzumab, another HER2-directed monoclonal antibody, binds effectively to JIMT-1 cells.[51]

The related proteoglycan MUC1 also has been implicated as a mediator of primary trastuzumab resistance. Proteolytic cleavage of full-length MUC1 yields a cell surface-associated fragment termed MUC1*. BT-474 cells with acquired trastuzumab resistance exhibit greatly increased concentrations of MUC1*, and siRNA knockdown of MUC1*, or antibodies directed against MUC1* reverse-acquired trastuzumab resistance in BT-474 cells.[52] MUC1* apparently plays a similar role in primary trastuzumab resistance: primary trastuzumab-resistant ZR-75-30 and T47D cells express MUC1*, and either knockdown or antibody-mediated inhibition of MUC1* induce trastuzumab sensitivity in these cell lines. While MUC1* could potentially inhibit trastuzumab's association with HER2 via steric hindrance, MUC1* expression has been independently correlated with induction of mitogen activated protein kinase (MAPK) phosphorylation and also with cell survival and proliferation.[53,54] Therefore, the precise mechanism underlying MUC1*'s role in trastuzumab resistance remains unclear.

In addition to these associations with extracellular matrix and cell surface proteoglycans, cytosolic regulators of HER2 stability have been identified as critical mediators of primary trastuzumab resistance. HER2 was recently identified as a target of the cysteine protease calpain-1, and pharmacologic inhibition of calpain-1 was found to desensitize trastuzumab-sensitive cells (see Fig. 1, panel E).[55] This finding is novel and unanticipated, as calpain is known to couple to EGFR and Src signaling to enhance motility and transformation,[56] but in the case of HER2, calpain has been proposed to function as an signaling attenuator.[55]

Molecular chaperones also have been implicated in the development of primary trastuzumab resistance. For example, HSP90 is well known to regulate the stability of client proteins such as HER2, decreasing receptor turnover thereby potentiating HER2 signaling (see Fig. 1, panel E).[57] Consequently, pharmacologic inhibition of HSP90 has become an area of intense study for overcoming trastuzumab resistance. In this regard, the cleaved tumorigenic HER2 fragment, p95HER2, has been identified as a client protein of the molecular chaperone HSP90, and trastuzumab-resistant breast cancer cells expressing p95HER2 exhibit growth inhibition by the HSP90 inhibitors *in vitro* and *in vivo*.[58,59] Although these studies do not directly identify HSP90 as a mediator of primary trastuzumab resistance, they do validate HSP90 as a potential therapeutic target in trastuzumab-resistant patients. Furthermore, expression of an HSP90-interacting protein, DARPP-32 and its truncated isoform tDarpp, also have been shown to confer primary trastuzumab resistance in BT474 and SKBR-3 cells.[60] Although DARPP-32 and tDarpp form a complex with HER2 and HSP90 in trastuzumab-resistant breast cancer cells,[61] the function of DARPP-32 and tDarpp in this complex has not yet been examined.

Activation of downstream effectors and signal crosstalk

In a small cohort of stage II/III breast cancer patients, Yonemori and colleagues[62] have found an association between responsiveness to neo-adjuvant therapy (trastuzumab plus chemotherapy) and tumor HER2 expression, but not with phosphatase and tensin homolog (PTEN), p53, estrogen receptor, progesterone receptor, or activated Akt expression. In contrast, Nagata and colleagues[63] have proposed that PTEN-deficiency in primary breast tumors from patients later treated with trastuzumab (for recurrent disease) is correlated with poor response to therapy. In support of this finding, Migliaccio and colleagues[64] have reported that patients treated with neoadjuvant trastuzumab plus docetaxel therapy who exhibit low tumor PTEN expression or *PIK3CA* mutations are less likely to respond to neoadjuvant

therapy. However, low PTEN expression or *PIK3CA* mutation status does not predict responsiveness to neoadjuvant lapatinib therapy, suggesting an involvement of EGFR signaling and/or differential responsiveness of tumors to HER2-directed tyrosine kinase inhibitors versus therapeutic antibodies. Gori and colleagues[65] further reported decreased survival in response to trastuzumab therapy among patients with elevated levels of phosphorylated MAPK. Related *in vitro* studies using panels of breast cancer cell lines have identified phosphatidylinositol 3-kinase (PI3K) expression,[66] low PTEN expression,[66] Akt phosphorylation,[66] and S6K phosphorylation[67] as potential mediators of primary trastuzumab resistance in breast cancer; the role of *PIK3CA* mutation in primary trastuzumab resistance *in vitro* is supported by Katoaka and colleagues[67] but not by Koninki and colleagues.[68]

Recent studies also have implicated protein kinase A (PKA) signaling as a mediator of trastuzumab resistance. Treatment with the adenylyl cyclase agonist forskolin confers partial resistance to trastuzumab-mediated survival signaling inhibition (i.e., Akt activation) in trastuzumab-sensitive cells, and siRNA-mediated knockdown of the PKA-negative regulator PKA-RIIα also confers partial resistance to trastuzumab-mediated growth inhibition of BT474 cells.[69] Additionally, Vegran and colleagues[43] have identified upregulation of *PRKACA*, the gene encoding the catalytic α-subunit of PKA, as an upregulated gene product in patients with trastuzumab-resistant breast cancer. Among the small cluster of upregulated gene products in patients with primary trastuzumab-resistant breast cancer identified by Vegran and colleagues are several cell signaling and cell cycle regulators, including the WEE1 homologue, protein phosphatase 2A, and CDC14A.[43]

Finally, Cheng and colleagues[70] have demonstrated a role for the well-known protein synthesis regulator, eEF-2 kinase, in primary trastuzumab resistance. siRNA-mediated knockdown of eEF-2 kinase, a negative regulator of eukaryotic elongation factor-2, sensitizes MCF7 and MDA-MB-468 cells to trastuzumab.

Since numerous factors regulate PKA activity, cell cycle progression, and protein synthesis, these findings provide further evidence of the complexity of primary trastuzumab resistance (see Fig. 1, panel F).

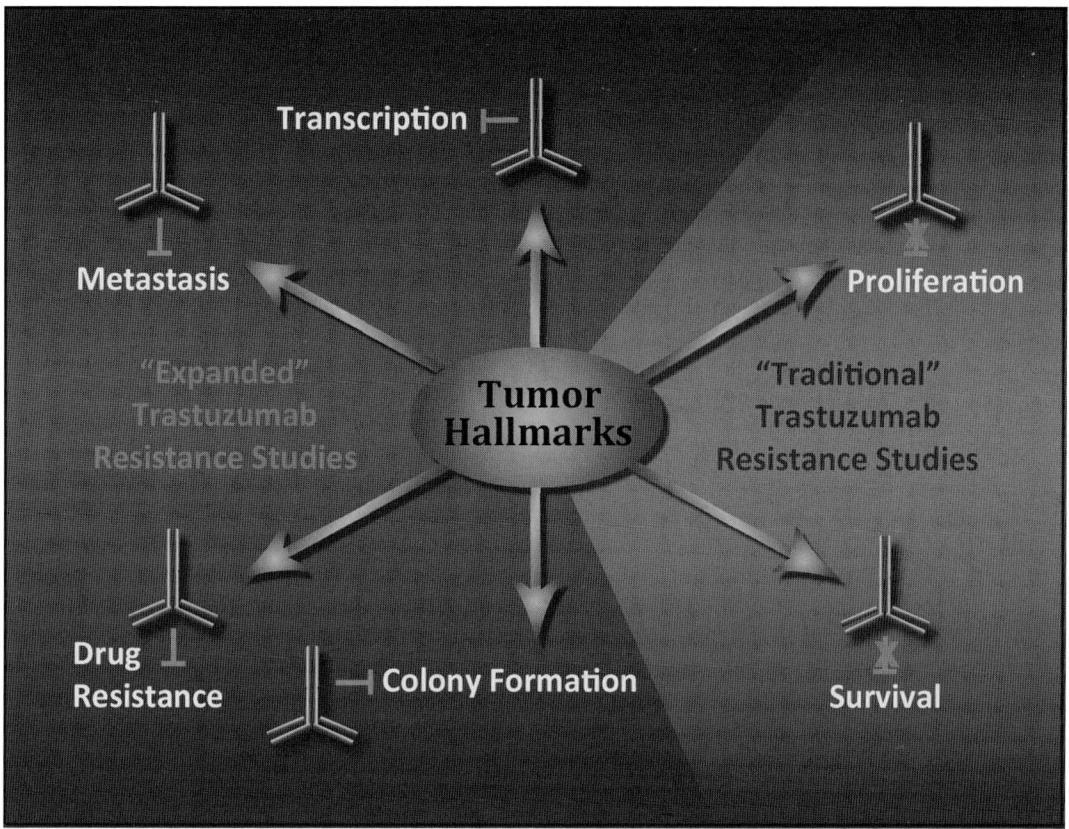

Figure 2. Models of primary trastuzumab resistance. The majority of studies examining the action of trastuzumab (and subsequent *acquired* resistance to trastuzumab) have focused on studies of cell proliferation and survival (i.e., "traditional" trastuzumab resistance). As summarized in this review, emerging evidence suggests we need to consider a more expansive definition of trastuzumab action, by including diverse functional assays for biological endpoints, such as migration and metastasis, anchorage dependence, patterns of gene expression, and the influence of trastuzumab on cell responses to other biologically targeted therapeutics. Multiple studies show that trastuzumab may influence all of these diverse cell phenotypes without directly influencing tumor cell proliferation or survival.

Cell: extracellular matrix interactions

Information from studies using carcinoma-derived cell lines is limited by the artificial and highly selected nature of these *in vitro* models. Nowhere is this limitation more apparent than in studies on the cell's microenvironment, including those of cell/matrix and cell/tissue interactions. The vast majority of *in vitro* studies using carcinoma-derived cell lines use rigid tissue culture plastic as an adherence medium. One exception, however is a recent study by Weigelt and colleagues,[71] who studied the influence of the microenvironment on trastuzumab resistance (see Fig. 1, panel G) using matrix-coated substrates. When grown on a laminin-rich matrix versus untreated plastic, SKBR-3 cells are, remarkably, not growth inhibited by trastuzumab.

This laminin matrix-mediated trastuzumab resistance was transduced through interactions between laminin and integrins, as evidenced by a reversal of trastuzumab resistance when SKBR-3 cells were treated with a β1-integrin inhibitory antibody.[71] In support of this concept, *LAMA3*, encoding laminin α3, has been identified as part of a gene profile upregulated among patients with primary trastuzumab-resistant breast cancer.[43]

In further support of this provocative finding, a recent retrospective study of patients with metastatic HER2-positive breast cancer has shown that β1-integrin expression is inversely correlated with survival among patients treated with trastuzumab but not with other regimens.[72] Moreover, transfection of β1 integrin into SKBR3 cells renders these cells resistant to trastuzumab-mediated growth inhibition.[72] Related results have been reported in another *in vitro* model (ovarian cancer) of long-term trastuzumab treatment in which tensin and RhoB regulation of tumor cell morphology has been proposed as a mediator of trastuzumab resistance.[73]

Noncytostatic effects of trastuzumab

Inhibition of cell proliferation *in vitro*, or of tumor growth *in vivo* are typically used as measures of efficacy for biologically targeted therapeutics, and with good reason. However, other more subtle phenotypic changes involving alternative biological endpoints may be manifest following trastuzumab treatment, as summarized in Figure 2. Critically, some of these latent phenotypes may be clinically relevant. Identification of these novel phenotypes may, therefore, allow us to more effectively treat breast cancer patients in the future.

Trastuzumab mediates de novo sensitization to drugs, ligands, and radiation

Several reports have demonstrated that trastuzumab may render tumor cells sensitive to therapeutics, independent of tumor cell growth inhibition. We have demonstrated, using HER2-positive breast carcinoma cell lines not growth inhibited by trastuzumab, long-term trastuzumab treatment results in an increase in EGFR expression in three of five cell lines; all five cell lines also showed an increase in HER3 expression.[73] In this study, one cell line (MDA-MB-361) acquired sensitivity to the EGFR-targeted antibody cetuximab, and a second cell line (MDA-MB-453) acquired sensitivity to the EGFR small molecule inhibitor gefitinib. Although such cell lines are not precise surrogates for the study of early stage HER2-positive breast cancer, this is the first study to demonstrate that long-term trastuzumab treatment of primary resistant cells has unambiguous effects on the tumor cell phenotype independent of this drug's effect on cell proliferation. Subsequent studies demonstrating that primary trastuzumab-resistant ovarian and lung cancer cells cultured with either trastuzumab or gefitinib (respectively), can sensitize these cells to other HER-directed therapeutics,[74,75] suggesting that this pattern of drug-induced HER-axis "reprogramming" may be a common theme in primary resistance to EGFR/HER2-directed therapeutics.

Concomitantly, long-term trastuzumab treatment also influences HER ligand-mediated cell proliferation. We have preliminary data showing that long-term treatment with trastuzumab alters both epidermal growth factor (EGF) and heregulin-mediated proliferative responses, despite the lack of trastuzumab cell growth inhibition in these cells. Similarly, patterns of HER ligand (EGF and heregulin)-stimulated phosphorylation of HER receptors and Akt are markedly different in gefitinib-resistant lung cancer cells cultured long-term with gefitinib.[74] This altered growth factor/ligand response phenotype may be related to changes in the expression pattern of HER receptors; the number of cell lines used in this initial study was limited, and so the results of these studies will need to be expanded and confirmed.

Several reports indicate that trastuzumab induces *de novo* sensitization to other drugs, including sensitization of MDA-MB-453 cells to all-trans retinoic acid[76] and to the proteosome inhibitor bortezomib,[77] sensitization of KPL-4 and JIMT-1 cells to an immunomodulatory oligonucleotide toll-like receptor 9 agonist,[78] and as mentioned above, sensitization of JIMT-1 cells to antibodies directed against β1-integrin.[71] As some of these drugs are in various stages of clinical testing, the prospect of rapidly integrating this new information into the design of innovative clinical studies merits consideration.

One recent study has demonstrated synergy between trastuzumab and the antidiabetic drug metformin. Although trastuzumab alone had no effect on the formation of JIMT-1 cell mammospheres *in vitro*, metformin, alone or in synergy with trastuzumab, inhibited mammosphere formation.[79] Metformin has previously been demonstrated as protective for the development of breast cancer,[80] and a phase II trial recently has opened to evaluate the efficacy of trastuzumab plus metformin as neoadjuvant therapy for patients with HER2-positive breast cancer.[81] As metformin exhibits pleiotropic effects on cells, the mechanism underlying metformin's synergy with trastuzumab is unclear, but may include 5′ adenosine monophosphate-activated protein kinase (AMPK) activation, cell cycle arrest, and/or metabolic alterations.[80]

Finally, Liang and colleagues[82] have shown that some trastuzumab-resistant breast cancer cells are sensitized to ionizing radiation following trastuzumab treatment. Induction of apoptosis was not observed in MDA-MB-453 or MCF7-HER2 cells following trastuzumab treatment, but synergistic induction of apoptosis was noted with trastuzumab and ionizing radiation; this synergism could be duplicated using the inhibitor LY294002, suggesting that trastuzumab treatment inhibits PI3K activity in MCF7-HER2 cells. Although the role of radiation therapy has been more limited in the treatment of breast cancer patients, the notion that drug priming of tumor cells prior to radiation treatment is one that has been exploited for the treatment of other adult solid tumors, and may be worth further consideration in breast cancer as well.

Colony formation, micrometastasis, and cytotoxicity

Barok and colleagues[83] recently have described another prime example of a nonproliferative effect of trastuzumab treatment. Established JIMT-1 tumors in a xenograft model are not significantly growth inhibited by trastuzumab. However, trastuzumab does effectively inhibit the level of circulating JIMT-1 tumor cells and distant micrometastases in this model,[84] likely through an immune-mediated mechanism, which may explain the observation cited above (i.e., concurrent trastuzumab treatment inhibits both the seeding and proliferation of JIMT-1 cells a xenograft model).[83] Similarly, KPL-4 cells, although not growth inhibited by trastuzumab *in vitro*, are growth inhibited by trastuzumab in a xenograft model only if trastuzumab has an intact FcγR.[85] UACC812 and UACC893 cells also are not growth inhibited by trastuzumab *in vitro*, but are sensitive to trastuzumab-mediated ADCC *in vitro*.[68]

In related studies, trastuzumab has been shown to inhibit soft agar colony formation of SUM-190 and HCC-202 cells *in vitro*, despite the failure of this drug to inhibit the growth of these cells when assayed in two-dimensional growth conditions.[66] Conversely, at least one cell line (UACC-732) that is modestly growth inhibited by trastuzumab in two-dimensional growth conditions is not growth inhibited by trastuzumab when cultured in soft agar colony.[66] Trastuzumab also has been shown to inhibit colony formation (on tissue culture plastic) of freshly dispersed T47D cells,[86] but not of cells already growing as a monolayer.[73] Remark-

ably, this inhibition of T47D colony formation can be reversed by induction of cyclin D1.[86] Although colony formation assays have long been used as a sensitive and stringent measure of cytotoxic activity, colony formation is also a measure of cell growth and plating (i.e., attachment) efficiency; therefore, interpretation of trastuzumab's mechanism of action in these studies is challenging. These studies remind us of the importance of selecting *in vitro* assays that allow us to more precisely distinguish between the oncogenic versus mitogenic aspects of HER-mediated signal transduction[87] during all phases of drug development and testing, as well as the importance of such distinctions in defining the mechanisms of primary trastuzumab resistance.

Altered expression and phosphorylation

One of the first indications of the complex relationship between trastuzumab sensitivity and changes in gene expression arose from studies on virally infected tumor-derived cell lines.[88] In particular, the MCF7 cell line expresses low levels of HER2, which can be induced by treatment with estradiol, and trastuzumab can inhibit expression of estrogen receptor alpha in this cell line.[89] Epstein-Barr Virus (EBV) infected MCF7 cells express elevated levels of HER2 and HER3, and EBV-infected (or *BARF0*-transfected) cells acquire *de novo* sensitivity to trastuzumab.[88] Together, these results highlight the complex relationship between viral infection and changes in gene expression, and the impact of such changes on responsiveness to trastuzumab.

In contrast, a few studies have demonstrated that trastuzumab can induce changes in gene expression without inhibiting cell proliferation. For example, both the MDA-MB-436 and MCF7 cell lines exhibit reproducible changes in the pattern of trastuzumab-induced gene expression (as measured by cDNA microarray), including changes in expression patterns of the FK506-binding protein, interleukin 2 receptor β, MUC2, plasminogen activator, kit, and fos.[90] Similarly, in JIMT-1 cells, trastuzumab treatment does not inhibit Akt phosphorylation, which is contrary to trastuzumab's effect on SKBR-3 cells; however, trastuzumab can downregulate MAPK phosphorylation in both of these cell lines.[91]

Although the potential biological and clinical significance of these *in vitro* studies on gene expression is intriguing, there is not yet a direct link between any of these observations and their relationship to primary trastuzumab resistance. These observations do, however, further underscore the apparent disconnect between the failure of trastuzumab to inhibit tumor cell growth and the ability of this drug to induce many important phenotypic changes in the tumor cell.

Summary and conclusions

Trastuzumab is unquestionably effective as a therapeutic for some patients with "HER2-positive" breast cancer. However, the mechanisms of primary trastuzumab resistance have yet to be thoroughly characterized, and a simple constellation of the mediators of primary trastuzumab resistance has not been identified. The results of the early studies in this field, summarized here, while compelling in their demonstration that primary trastuzumab resistance can be correlated with certain patterns of gene expression, need to be interpreted with caution and also require further validation in prospective clinical trials. Patient heterogeneity, treatment of patients with combinations of trastuzumab and other drugs, small population/cohort sizes, (most studies included <50 patients), methodological differences in retrospective versus prospective studies, tumor histological subtype (including primary vs. metastatic disease), and finally, the lack of external validation using independent patient populations, all limit our ability to extrapolate and generalize the findings from these studies across patient populations.

Despite these limitations, including the paucity of both clinically validated studies and adequate model systems, an important theme emerges from these studies: trastuzumab can induce important noncytostatic responses across model systems. Critically, some of these noncytostatic effects result in clinically significant phenotypic changes that may be useful in *de novo* sensitization of tumor cells to other drugs and/or treatment modalities. Moreover, these studies highlight the need to develop a better, comprehensive definition of resistance to trastuzumab and perhaps to other biologically targeted drugs that is consonant with the subtle but important phenotypic changes that may predictably be associated with exposure to biologically targeted therapeutics.

In conclusion, the unanticipated findings summarized here support the proposal that primary trastuzumab resistance should be defined us-ing metrics beyond those restricted to conventional measures of drug inhibition of tumor cell proliferation. Recognition of these more subtle trastuzumab-induced biological phenotypes may be useful in the development of improved methods of cancer patient treatment, through the identification of common, targetable mediators of resistance that will allow us to better exploit all aspects of trastuzumab's therapeutic potential.

Acknowledgments

Grant support: J.A.W. is supported by Susan G. Komen for the Cure and the Marsha Rivkin Center for Ovarian Cancer Research. N.J.M. is supported by NIH CA 79808 and a "Senior Women in Medicine Professorship" from Yale University School of Medicine. We thank Ms. Tayf Badri for her assistance in preparation of this review, Drs. Andre T. Baron and Karin Rodland for editorial comments, Drs. Murli Narayan and Lyndsay Harris for their contributions to these studies, and KJ Studios (www.kjstudios.com) for expert assistance with artwork presented here.

Conflicts of interest

The authors declare no conflicts of interest.

References

1. Allison, M. 2010. The HER2 testing conundrum. *Nat. Biotechnol.* **28:** 117–119.
2. Nahta, R., M.C. Hung & F.J. Esteva. 2004. The HER-2-targeting antibodies trastuzumab and pertuzumab synergistically inhibit the survival of breast cancer cells. *Cancer Res.* **64:** 2343–2346.
3. Arnould, L. *et al.* 2006. Trastuzumab-based treatment of HER2-positive breast cancer: an antibody-dependent cellular cytotoxicity mechanism? *Br. J. Cancer* **94:** 259–267.
4. Pegram, M. *et al.* 1999. Inhibitory effects of combinations of HER-2/neu antibody and chemotherapeutic agents used for treatment of human breast cancers. *Oncogene* **18:** 2241–2251.
5. Slamon, D.J. *et al.* 2001. Use of chemotherapy plus a monoclonal antibody against HER2 for metastatic breast cancer that overexpresses HER2. *N. Engl. J. Med.* **344:** 783–792.
6. Pupa, S.M. *et al.* 1993. The extracellular domain of the c-erbB-2 oncoprotein is released from tumor cells by proteolytic cleavage. *Oncogene* **8:** 2917–2923.
7. Zabrecky, J.R. *et al.* 1991. The extracellular domain of p185/neu is released from the surface of human breast carcinoma cells, SK-BR-3. *J. Biol. Chem.* **266:** 1716–1720.
8. Codony-Servat, J. *et al.* 1999. Cleavage of the HER2 ectodomain is a pervanadate-activable process that is inhibited by the tissue inhibitor of metalloproteases-1 in breast cancer cells. *Cancer Res.* **59:** 1196–1201.

9. Lafky, J.M. *et al.* 2008. Clinical implications of the ErbB/epidermal growth factor (EGF) receptor family and its ligands in ovarian cancer. *Biochim. Biophys. Acta* **1785:** 232–265.

10. Molina, M.A. *et al.* 2001. Trastuzumab (herceptin), a humanized anti-Her2 receptor monoclonal antibody, inhibits basal and activated Her2 ectodomain cleavage in breast cancer cells. *Cancer Res.* **61:** 4744–4749.

11. Christianson, T.A. *et al.* 1998. NH2-terminally truncated HER-2/neu protein: relationship with shedding of the extracellular domain and with prognostic factors in breast cancer. *Cancer Res.* **58:** 5123–5129.

12. Anido, J. *et al.* 2006. Biosynthesis of tumorigenic HER2 C-terminal fragments by alternative initiation of translation. *EMBO J.* **25:** 3234–3244.

13. Drebin, J.A. *et al.* 1985. Down-modulation of an oncogene protein product and reversion of the transformed phenotype by monoclonal antibodies. *Cell* **41:** 697–706.

14. Hurwitz, E. *et al.* 1995. Suppression and promotion of tumor growth by monoclonal antibodies to ErbB-2 differentially correlate with cellular uptake. *Proc. Natl. Acad. Sci. USA* **92:** 3353–3357.

15. Klapper, L.N. *et al.* 2000. Tumor-inhibitory antibodies to HER-2/ErbB-2 may act by recruiting c-Cbl and enhancing ubiquitination of HER-2. *Cancer Res.* **60:** 3384–3388.

16. Baselga, J. & S.M. Swain. 2009. Novel anticancer targets: revisiting ERBB2 and discovering ERBB3. *Nat. Rev. Cancer* **9:** 463–475.

17. Spector, N.L. & K.L. Blackwell. 2009. Understanding the mechanisms behind trastuzumab therapy for human epidermal growth factor receptor 2-positive breast cancer. *J. Clin. Oncol.* **27:** 5838–5847.

18. Pohlmann, P.R., I.A. Mayer & R. Mernaugh. 2009. Resistance to trastuzumab in breast cancer. *Clin. Cancer Res.* **15:** 7479–7491.

19. Harris, L.N. *et al.* 2007. Predictors of resistance to preoperative trastuzumab and vinorelbine for HER2-positive early breast cancer. *Clin. Cancer Res.* **13:** 1198–1207.

20. Wolff, A.C. *et al.* 2007. American Society of Clinical Oncology/College of American Pathologists guideline recommendations for human epidermal growth factor receptor 2 testing in breast cancer. *J. Clin. Oncol.* **25:** 118–145.

21. Romond, E.H. *et al.* 2005. Trastuzumab plus adjuvant chemotherapy for operable HER2-positive breast cancer. *N. Engl. J. Med.* **353:** 1673–1684.

22. Doherty, J.K. *et al.* 1999. The HER-2/neu receptor tyrosine kinase gene encodes a secreted autoinhibitor. *Proc. Natl. Acad. Sci. USA* **96:** 10869–10874.

23. Scott, G.K. *et al.* 1993. A truncated intracellular HER2/neu receptor produced by alternative RNA processing affects growth of human carcinoma cells. *Mol. Cell Biol.* **13:** 2247–2257.

24. Pedersen, K. *et al.* 2009. A naturally occurring HER2 carboxy-terminal fragment promotes mammary tumor growth and metastasis. *Mol. Cell Biol.* **29:** 3319–3331.

25. Scaltriti, M. *et al.* 2007. Expression of p95HER2, a truncated form of the HER2 receptor, and response to anti-HER2 therapies in breast cancer. *J. Natl. Cancer Inst.* **99:** 628–638.

26. Molina, M.A. *et al.* 2002. NH(2)-terminal truncated HER-2 protein but not full-length receptor is associated with nodal metastasis in human breast cancer. *Clin. Cancer Res.* **8:** 347–353.

27. Saez, R. *et al.* 2006. p95HER-2 predicts worse outcome in patients with HER-2-positive breast cancer. *Clin. Cancer Res.* **12:** 424–431.

28. Sperinde, J. *et al.* 2010. Quantitation of p95HER2 in paraffin sections using a p95-specific antibody and correlation with outcome in a cohort of trastuzumab-treated breast cancer patients. *Clin. Cancer Res.* **16:** 4226–4235.

29. Brodowicz, T. *et al.* 1997. Soluble HER-2/neu neutralizes biologic effects of anti-HER-2/neu antibody on breast cancer cells in vitro. *Int. J. Cancer* **73:** 875–879.

30. Ghedini, G.C. *et al.* 2010. Shed HER2 extracellular domain in HER2-mediated tumor growth and in Trastuzumab susceptibility. *J. Cell Physiol.*

31. Ali, S.M. *et al.* 2008. Serum HER-2/neu and relative resistance to trastuzumab-based therapy in patients with metastatic breast cancer. *Cancer* **113:** 1294–1301.

32. Lennon, S. *et al.* 2009. Utility of serum HER2 extracellular domain assessment in clinical decision making: pooled analysis of four trials of trastuzumab in metastatic breast cancer. *J. Clin. Oncol.* **27:** 1685–1693.

33. Witzel, I. *et al.* 2010. Monitoring serum HER2 levels during neoadjuvant trastuzumab treatment within the GeparQuattro trial. *Breast Cancer Res. Treat.* **123:** 437–445.

34. Arnould, L. *et al.* 2007. Pathologic complete response to trastuzumab-based neoadjuvant therapy is related to the level of HER-2 amplification. *Clin. Cancer Res.* **13:** 6404–6409.

35. Ginestier, C. *et al.* 2007. ERBB2 phosphorylation and trastuzumab sensitivity of breast cancer cell lines. *Oncogene* **26:** 7163–7169.

36. Weinstein, I.B. 2002. Cancer. Addiction to oncogenes—the Achilles heal of cancer. *Science* **297:** 63–64.

37. Narayan, M. *et al.* 2009. Trastuzumab-induced HER reprogramming in "resistant" breast carcinoma cells. *Cancer Res.* In Press.

38. Dua, R. *et al.* 2010. EGFR over-expression and activation in high HER2, ER negative breast cancer cell line induces trastuzumab resistance. *Breast Cancer Res. Treat.* **122:** 685–697.

39. Yotsumoto, F. *et al.* 2010. HB-EGF orchestrates the complex signals involved in triple-negative and trastuzumab-resistant breast cancer. *Int. J. Cancer.* In Press.

40. Yonemori, K. *et al.* 2010. Immunohistochemical expression of HER1, HER3, and HER4 in HER2-positive breast cancer patients treated with trastuzumab-containing neoadjuvant chemotherapy. *J. Surg. Oncol.* **101:** 222–227.

41. Jerome, L. *et al.* 2006. Recombinant human insulin-like growth factor binding protein 3 inhibits growth of human epidermal growth factor receptor-2-overexpressing breast tumors and potentiates herceptin activity in vivo. *Cancer Res.* **66:** 7245–7252.

42. Lu, Y. *et al.* 2001. Insulin-like growth factor-I receptor signaling and resistance to trastuzumab (Herceptin). *J. Natl. Cancer Inst.* **93:** 1852–1857.

43. Vegran, F. *et al.* 2009. Gene expression profile and response to trastuzumab-docetaxel-based treatment in breast carcinoma. *Br. J. Cancer* **101:** 1357–1364.

44. Zhuang, G. *et al.* 2010. Elevation of receptor tyrosine kinase EphA2 mediates resistance to trastuzumab therapy. *Cancer Res.* **70:** 299–308.

45. Martin, K.J. *et al.* 2008. Prognostic breast cancer signature identified from 3D culture model accurately predicts clinical outcome across independent datasets. *PLoS ONE* **3:** e2994.

46. Fournier, M.V. *et al.* 2006. Gene expression signature in organized and growth-arrested mammary acini predicts good outcome in breast cancer. *Cancer Res.* **66:** 7095–7102.

47. Cavalloni, G. *et al.* 2008. Granulocyte-colony stimulating factor upregulates ErbB2 expression on breast cancer cell lines and converts primary resistance to trastuzumab. *Anticancer Drugs* **19:** 689–696.

48. Mocanu, M.M. *et al.* 2005. Associations of ErbB2, beta1-integrin and lipid rafts on Herceptin (Trastuzumab) resistant and sensitive tumor cell lines. *Cancer Lett.* **227:** 201–212.

49. Palyi-Krekk, Z. *et al.* 2007. Hyaluronan-induced masking of ErbB2 and CD44-enhanced trastuzumab internalisation in trastuzumab resistant breast cancer. *Eur. J. Cancer* **43:** 2423–2433.

50. Price-Schiavi, S.A. *et al.* 2002. Rat Muc4 (sialomucin complex) reduces binding of anti-ErbB2 antibodies to tumor cell surfaces, a potential mechanism for herceptin resistance. *Int. J. Cancer* **99:** 783–791.

51. Nagy, P. *et al.* 2005. Decreased accessibility and lack of activation of ErbB2 in JIMT-1, a herceptin-resistant, MUC4-expressing breast cancer cell line. *Cancer Res.* **65:** 473–482.

52. Fessler, S.P. *et al.* 2009. MUC1* is a determinant of trastuzumab (Herceptin) resistance in breast cancer cells. *Breast Cancer Res. Treat.* **118:** 113–124.

53. Hikita, S.T. *et al.* 2008. MUC1* mediates the growth of human pluripotent stem cells. *PLoS ONE* **3:** e3312.

54. Mahanta, S. *et al.* 2008. A minimal fragment of MUC1 mediates growth of cancer cells. *PLoS ONE* **3:** e2054.

55. Kulkarni, S. *et al.* 2009. Calpain regulates sensitivity to trastuzumab and survival in HER2-positive breast cancer. *Oncogene* **29:** 1339–1350.

56. Carragher, N.O. & M.C. Frame. 2002. Calpain: a role in cell transformation and migration. *Int. J. Biochem. Cell Biol.* **34:** 1539–1543.

57. Citri, A., B.S. Kochupurakkal & Y. Yarden. 2004. The achilles heel of ErbB-2/HER2: regulation by the Hsp90 chaperone machine and potential for pharmacological intervention. *Cell Cycle* **3:** 51–60.

58. Chandarlapaty, S. *et al.* 2010. Inhibitors of HSP90 block p95-HER2 signaling in Trastuzumab-resistant tumors and suppress their growth. *Oncogene* **29:** 325–334.

59. Leow, C.C. *et al.* 2009. Antitumor efficacy of IPI-504, a selective heat shock protein 90 inhibitor against human epidermal growth factor receptor 2-positive human xenograft models as a single agent and in combination with trastuzumab or lapatinib. *Mol Cancer Ther.* **8:** 2131–2141.

60. Hamel, S. *et al.* 2010. Both t-Darpp and DARPP-32 can cause resistance to trastuzumab in breast cancer cells and are frequently expressed in primary breast cancers. *Breast Cancer Res. Treat.* **120:** 47–57.

61. Belkhiri, A. *et al.* 2008. Expression of t-DARPP mediates trastuzumab resistance in breast cancer cells. *Clin. Cancer Res.* **14:** 4564–4571.

62. Yonemori, K. *et al.* 2009. Immunohistochemical expression of PTEN and phosphorylated Akt are not correlated with clinical outcome in breast cancer patients treated with trastuzumab-containing neo-adjuvant chemotherapy. *Med. Oncol.* **26:** 344–349.

63. Nagata, Y. *et al.* 2004. PTEN activation contributes to tumor inhibition by trastuzumab, and loss of PTEN predicts trastuzumab resistance in patients. *Cancer Cell* **6:** 117–127.

64. Migliaccio, I. *et al.* 2008. PI3 kinase activation and response to trastuzumab or lapatinib in HER-2 overexpressing locally advanced breast cancer (LABC). In Proceedings of the *San Antonio Breast Cancer Symposium: Abstract 34*. San Antonio, TX.

65. Gori, S. *et al.* 2009. EGFR, pMAPK, pAkt and PTEN status by immunohistochemistry: correlation with clinical outcome in HER2-positive metastatic breast cancer patients treated with trastuzumab. *Ann. Oncol.* **20:** 648–654.

66. O'Brien, N.A. *et al.* 2010. Activated phosphoinositide 3-kinase/AKT signaling confers resistance to trastuzumab but not lapatinib. *Mol. Cancer Ther.* **9:** 1489–1502.

67. Kataoka, Y. *et al.* 2010. Association between gain-of-function mutations in PIK3CA and resistance to HER2-targeted agents in HER2-amplified breast cancer cell lines. *Ann. Oncol.* **21:** 255–262.

68. Koninki, K. *et al.* 2010. Multiple molecular mechanisms underlying trastuzumab and lapatinib resistance in JIMT-1 breast cancer cells. *Cancer Lett.* **294:** 211–219.

69. Gu, L. *et al.* 2009. Protein kinase A activation confers resistance to trastuzumab in human breast cancer cell lines. *Clin. Cancer Res.* **15:** 7196–7206.

70. Cheng, Y. *et al.* 2010. Cytoprotective effect of the elongation factor-2 kinase-mediated autophagy in breast cancer cells subjected to growth factor inhibition. *PLoS ONE* **5:** e9715.

71. Weigelt, B. *et al.* 2009. HER2 signaling pathway activation and response of breast cancer cells to HER2-targeting agents is dependent strongly on the 3D microenvironment. *Breast Cancer Res. Treat.* **122:** 35–43.

72. Lesniak, D. *et al.* 2009. Beta1-integrin circumvents the antiproliferative effects of trastuzumab in human epidermal growth factor receptor-2-positive breast cancer. *Cancer Res.* **69:** 8620–8628.

73. Delord, J.P. *et al.* 2010. Trastuzumab induced in vivo tissue remodelling associated in vitro with inhibition of the active forms of AKT and PTEN and RhoB induction in an ovarian carcinoma model. *Br. J. Cancer* **103:** 61–72.

74. Jain, A. *et al.* 2010. HER kinase axis receptor dimer partner switching occurs in response to EGFR tyrosine kinase inhibition despite failure to block cellular proliferation. *Cancer Res.* **70:** 1989–1999.

75. Wilken, J.A., K.T. Webster & N.J. Maihle. 2010. Trastuzumab sensitizes ovarian cancer cells to EGFR-targeted therapeutics. *J. Ovarian Res.* **3:** 7.

76. Tari, A.M. *et al.* 2002. Her2/neu induces all-trans retinoic acid (ATRA) resistance in breast cancer cells. *Oncogene* **21:** 5224–5232.

77. Cardoso, F. *et al.* 2006. Bortezomib (PS-341, Velcade) increases the efficacy of trastuzumab (Herceptin) in HER-2-positive breast cancer cells in a synergistic manner. *Mol. Cancer Ther.* **5:** 3042–3051.

78. Damiano, V. *et al.* 2009. A novel toll-like receptor 9 agonist cooperates with trastuzumab in trastuzumab-resistant breast tumors through multiple mechanisms of action. *Clin. Cancer Res.* **15:** 6921–6930.

79. Vazquez-Martin, A. *et al.* 2010. The anti-diabetic drug metformin suppresses self-renewal and proliferation of trastuzumab-resistant tumor-initiating breast cancer stem cells. *Breast Cancer Res. Treat.* In Press.

80. Papanas, N., E. Maltezos & D.P. Mikhailidis. 2010. Metformin and cancer: licence to heal? *Expert Opin. Investig. Drugs* **19:** 913–917.

81. Martin-Castillo, B. *et al.* 2010. Incorporating the antidiabetic drug metformin in HER2-positive breast cancer treated with neo-adjuvant chemotherapy and trastuzumab: an ongoing clinical-translational research experience at the Catalan Institute of Oncology. *Ann. Oncol.* **21:** 187–189.

82. Liang, K. *et al.* 2003. Sensitization of breast cancer cells to radiation by trastuzumab. *Mol. Cancer Ther.* **2:** 1113–1120.

83. Barok, M. *et al.* 2007. Trastuzumab causes antibody-dependent cellular cytotoxicity-mediated growth inhibition of submacroscopic JIMT-1 breast cancer xenografts despite intrinsic drug resistance. *Mol. Cancer Ther.* **6:** 2065–2072.

84. Barok, M. *et al.* 2008. Trastuzumab decreases the number of circulating and disseminated tumor cells despite trastuzumab resistance of the primary tumor. *Cancer Lett.* **260:** 198–208.

85. Junttila, T.T. *et al.* 2010. Superior in vivo efficacy of afucosylated trastuzumab in the treatment of HER2-amplified breast cancer. *Cancer Res.* **70:** 4481–4489.

86. Wu, K. *et al.* 2002. Flavopiridol and trastuzumab synergistically inhibit proliferation of breast cancer cells: association with selective cooperative inhibition of cyclin D1-dependent kinase and Akt signaling pathways. *Mol. Cancer Ther.* **1:** 695–706.

87. Boerner, J.L., A. Danielsen & N.J. Maihle. 2003. Ligand-independent oncogenic signaling by the epidermal growth factor receptor: v-ErbB as a paradigm. *Exp. Cell Res.* **284:** 111–121.

88. Lin, J.H. *et al.* 2007. Dysregulation of HER2/HER3 signaling axis in Epstein-Barr virus-infected breast carcinoma cells. *J. Virol.* **81:** 5705–5713.

89. Chang, C.J. *et al.* 2006. Modulation of HER2 expression by ferulic acid on human breast cancer MCF7 cells. *Eur. J. Clin. Invest.* **36:** 588–596.

90. Kauraniemi, P. *et al.* 2004. Effects of Herceptin treatment on global gene expression patterns in HER2-amplified and nonamplified breast cancer cell lines. *Oncogene* **23:** 1010–1013.

91. Tanner, M. *et al.* 2004. Characterization of a novel cell line established from a patient with Herceptin-resistant breast cancer. *Mol. Cancer Ther.* **3:** 1585–1592.

Ann. N.Y. Acad. Sci. ISSN 0077-8923

ANNALS OF THE NEW YORK ACADEMY OF SCIENCES

Issue: *Toward Personalized Medicine for Cancer*

Advancing personalized cancer therapy by detection and characterization of circulating carcinoma cells

Sabine Riethdorf and Klaus Pantel

Institute of Tumor Biology, University Medical Center Hamburg-Eppendorf, Hamburg, Germany

Address for correspondence: Klaus Pantel, M.D., Ph.D., Institute of Tumor Biology, University Medical Center Hamburg Eppendorf, Martinistr. 52, D-20246 Hamburg, Germany. pantel@uke.uni-hamburg.de

Early dissemination, blood circulation, or homing of single tumor cells in bone marrow and other organs is usually undetectable at primary diagnosis, even by high resolution imaging technologies. However, ultrasensitive approaches now enable the detection of "occult" tumor cells. Many researchers are currently focusing on circulating tumor cells (CTC) in peripheral blood, and several publications have described associations of CTC in patients with metastatic cancer and worse prognosis. However, evidence has emerged that the currently used detection methods lack sensitivity or specificity to track all CTC, especially those that have lost characteristic epithelial features. Therefore, new developments in this field are of utmost interest and will be reviewed here. Moreover, molecular CTC analysis will provide insights into the selection of tumor cells and resistance mechanisms in patients undergoing systemic therapies. This information might support assessing individual prognosis, stratifying patients at risk to systemic therapies, and monitoring therapeutic efficacy.

Keywords: solid tumors; circulating tumor cells; peripheral blood; disseminated tumor cells; bone marrow; prognosis; cancer therapy

Introduction

The prognosis of carcinoma patients even with small primary tumors is still limited by metastatic relapse frequently occurring years after diagnosis and complete resection of the primary tumors. This is caused by minimal residual disease (MRD) and the presence of single disseminated or circulating tumor cells (CTC) undetectable even by high resolution imaging technologies. To identify these rare cells in the bone marrow, lymph nodes, or blood, sensitive and specific assays have been developed.[1,2]

Bone marrow, easily accessible by aspiration through the iliac crest, plays the most prominent role among the distant organs as an indicator organ for MRD. Moreover, bone marrow appears to be a common homing organ for disseminated tumor cells derived from carcinomas of different organs,[3] and also might be a reservoir for disseminated tumor cells with the capacity to re-enter primary tumor sites, thus contributing to the development of local recurrences.[4] For longitudinal controls and long-term observation of cancer patients, sequential analyses are pivotal; therefore, many research groups are currently evaluating the clinical utility of analysis for CTC in peripheral blood to replace analysis of bone marrow for assessment of prognosis and monitoring of systemic therapy.[5]

Although a number of new innovative technologies to improve methods for detecting CTC, with extraordinarily high sensitivity, have recently been presented, including CTC microchips, filtration, quantitative RT-PCR, and progress in microscopic approaches, specificity and utility of these methods in large clinical studies have still to be demonstrated.[2]

Previous findings suggest that DTC/CTC are able to survive chemotherapy and radiation and to persist in a dormant nonproliferating state over many years.[6,7] Targeted anticancer therapies that are more effective than current therapies and less harmful to normal cells are specifically aimed to stop growth and kill these rare tumor cells. Currently, the decision for a targeted therapy of an individual patient is

doi: 10.1111/j.1749-6632.2010.05779.x

 Ann. N.Y. Acad. Sci. 1210 (2010) 66–77 © 2010 New York Academy of Sciences.

normally made by analyzing the primary tumor for the expression of a specific molecular target. However, this is often hampered by the heterogeneity and plasticity of individual tumor cells to differentially adapt to certain growth conditions. This article will focus on ways to detect and further characterize individual CTCs as a "liquid biopsy," to help identify therapeutic targets that might contribute to the development of improved individualized, targeted treatments of patients, and might provide the potential to monitor systemic tumor cell dissemination in bone marrow and blood.

Improvement in detection of CTC/DTC

To detect CTC, one faces three major problems: (a) the extraordinarily low number of cells in the background of normal blood cells (10^{-6}), (b) the lack of common tumor cell-specific markers applicable for CTC screening, and (c) heterogeneity and plasticity of CTC, with subpopulations that have lost characteristic epithelial features. Due to the extremely low frequency of CTC, several methods for the enrichment of tumor cells from peripheral blood have been developed, including density gradient centrifugation, immunomagnetic bead separation (either by antibodies against epithelial surface antigens as surrogate markers for epithelial tumor cells (positive selection) or depletion of CD45-positive cells in a negative selection), FACS sorting, and filtration based on the different sizes of tumor and normal blood cells.[1,8] A variety of methods to screen the peripheral blood for CTCs after enrichment has also been established: cytometric/immunological approaches, comprising a manifold of different methods (Table 1), and molecular approaches based on characterization of DNA or RNA.[1,9]

Detection by immunocytochemistry[3,9] not only enables the characterization of both cell size and shape (as well as the nucleus-plasma relation of each individual event thereby excluding several blood cells with illegitimate or weak expression of the protein of interest) but also allows the identification of the cellular localization of a specific immunoreaction. Because of the absence of tumor-specific target antigens in most tumor cells, epithelium-specific antigens such as cytoskeleton-associated cytokeratins, surface adhesion molecules, and growth factor receptors are still the markers of choice for the detection of CTC.[1,9] To circumvent the problem of strongly varying detection of DTC/CTC in cancer patients, a consensus concept for detecting and enriching DTC in bone marrow that also can be applied for the identification of CTC has been proposed, including criteria to evaluate morphology and staining results after automatic microscopic screening.[10] Further progress towards a standardized method for CTC detection in the peripheral blood was reached through the introduction of the CellSearch system, an automated enrichment and immunostaining device that has been cleared by the U.S. Food and Drug Administration for the detection of CTC in patients with metastatic breast, colon, and prostate cancer.[11–15] Since the CellSearch system is strongly dependent on detection of epithelial cell adhesion molecule (EpCAM) and cytokeratin expression, CTC negative for the expression of these epithelial characteristics, such as normal-like breast cancer, will not be recognized.[16] That the inability to detect CTC in a higher number is limited by technical difficulties as well as the low frequency of CTC was recently be shown by Lalmahomed and colleagues, who demonstrated that higher CTC numbers can be detected with the CellSearch system when using 30 mL instead of 7.5 mL blood.[17] On the other hand, Flores and colleagues reported that using the CellSearch Profile kit (instead of the CellSearch Epithelial kit) resulted in a significant improvement in isolating, and thus characterizing, CTC.[18] Interestingly, combined use of anti-EpCAM and anti-CD146 antibodies for CTC enrichment is likely to improve CTC detection in breast cancer patients.[19] Furthermore, interpretation of images obtained by the CellSearch system is intensively discussed, and Coumans and colleagues demonstrated that all circulating $EpCAM^+CK^+CD45^-$ objects might be predictive for overall survival in castration-resistant prostate cancer.[20]

Most immunocytochemical approaches require fixation steps, which excludes subsequent expression analysis and functional studies. A challenging and important prerequisite for functional testing is the isolation of viable DTC/CTC. Progress into this direction is derived from the introduction of the EPISPOT (epithelial immunospot) technique, allowing the detection of only viable CTC/DTC by their ability to secrete individual proteins after short-term culture. Applying this approach, Muc-1 and/or CK19-secreting DTC could

Table 1. Manifold of immunological methods for DTC/CTC detection

Approach	Source/volume	Carcinoma patients analyzed	Enrichment	Detection	Important notes
ACIS® Ariol® Automated scanning of chromogenic immunostainings	BM/blood	Breast, prostate, colorectal, and others	Density gradient centrifugation, MACS®	Positive markers: CK Negative control: MOPC-21 Nucleus: hemalaun	Enrichment independent of the expression of specific markers, morphological evaluation of DTC/CTC feasible[10]
CellSearch® system	Blood/ 7.5 mL	Breast, colorectal, prostate cancer, lung, urinary bladder, and others	EpCAM-Ab coupled ferrofluid, (CD146[19]-Ab coupled ferrofluid)	Positive marker: CK Negative marker: CD45 Nucleus: DAPI	Semi-automated system with FDA approval for metastatic breast, colon and prostate cancer[11-20]
EPISPOT assay	Blood, BM/ 10 mL	Breast, colorectal, prostate and thyroid cancer	Depletion of CD45+ cells	Secretion of proteins:CK19, MUC1, Cath-D (breast); CK19 (colon); PSA (prostate); TG (thyroid)	Detection of viable epithelial secreting-cells; unbiased enrichment independent of CTC/DTC phenotype[21]
CAM Assay	Blood, 3 mL	Breast, prostate, ovarian	Invasion and digestion of cell adhesion matrix	Positive marker: CK 4,5,6,8, 10,13, and 18 Negative marker: CD45	Detection of viable epithelial cells that bind, invade, and ingest CAM[23]
CTC-chip microchip	Blood/0.9 mL	NSCLC, pancreatic, breast, prostate, colorectal	EpCAM-Ab-coupled microposts	Positive marker: CK Negative marker: CD45 Nucleus: DAPI	High detection rate (approx. 100%) even in M_0-patients warrants further investigations on assay specificity[29-31]
Laser scanning cytometry Maintrac®	Blood, BM/ 10 mL	Breast, lung	RBC lysis	Positive marker: EpCAM, negative marker: CD45	High incidence of positive events up to 3 logs higher CTC counts than those obtained with other techniques warrants further investigations on assay specificity[34]
Ikoniscope® imaging system	Blood/1 mL	Prostate, colorectal, ovarian	Ficoll-Isopaque or filtration with track-etched membranes	Positive markers: EpCAM, CK7/8 PSA (prostate only) FISH: chromosomes 7 and 8 Nucleus: DAPI	Two epithelial specific Abs and FISH to detect chromosomal abnormalities in CTC[36]
Ariol® system Scanning of fluorescent immunostaining scanning)	Blood/7.5 mL	Breast	RBC lysis, then CK-Ab + EpCAM-Ab coupled microbeads	Positive markers: CK8, 18, 19 Negative marker: CD45 Nucleus: DAPI	Detection of EpCAM+ and EpCAM− CTC[35]

Continued

Table 1. *Continued*

Approach	Source/volume	Carcinoma patients analyzed	Enrichment	Detection	Important notes
MagSweeper	Blood/9 mL	Breast	EpCAM-Ab immunomagnetic cell separation (Dynabeads)	Gene expression profiling	Isolated cells are easily accessible and can be extracted individually on the basis of their physical characteristics to deplete any cells nonspecifically bound to beads; CTC enriched by 10^8-fold from blood[33]
Fibre-optic array scanning technology (FAST)	Blood/10 mL	Breast	No enrichment	Positive marker: CK	Scanning instrument using fiber-optic array scanning technology (FAST) that can locate CTC at a rate that is 500-times faster than ADM with comparable sensitivity and improved specificity; no purification and enrichment step required; 98% sensitivity[37]
Multiparameter flow cytometry	Blood/20 mL	Breast	Ficoll density gradient centrifugation	Positive marker: EpCAM, CK8, 18, 19 Negative marker: CD45	Sensitivity limit of 10^{-5}, higher specificity than RT-PCR[28]

EpCAM = epithelial cell adhesion molecule; Ab = antibody; CK = cytokeratin; DAPI = 4′,6-Diamidino-2-phenylindole; EPIS-POT = EPIthelial immunoSPOT; BM = bone marrow; MUC1 = mucine 1; Cath-D = cathepsin D; PSA = prostate specific antigen; TG = thyroglobulin; CTC = circulating tumor cells; NSCLC = nonsmall-cell lung cancer; RBC = red blood cells; FISH = fluorescent *in situ* hybridization; MOPC-21, mineral oil induced PlasmaCytoma-21; DAPI = 4′,6-diamidin-2′-phenylindoldihydrochlorid; MACS = magnetic cell separation; CAM = cell adhesion matrix; ADM = automated digital microscopy.

be demonstrated in bone marrow samples of breast cancer patients with (90%) and without (50%) metastases.[21] The detection of full-length CK19-expressing cells by this technique correlated with the presence of overt metastasis and a reduced survival.[22] A method that enriches viable CTC based on their unique ability to invade and ingest a cell adhesion matrix (CAM assay) was recently presented; this assay allows for distinguishing CTC from normal and dead cells, which are unable to bind, invade, and ingest CAM. Fluorescently labeled CAM fragments within CTC that are co-immunostained with antiepithelial antigen-specific antibodies have been identified in blood samples from carcinoma patients.[23] An additional new approach to visually detect live human CTC among millions of peripheral blood leukocytes, using a telomerase-specific replication-selective adenovirus expressing GFP (TelomeScan), was presented last year.[24] Upon incubation with tumor cells, the virus is only able to replicate in cancer cells and thereby incorporates GFP, which is then used to detect the cells by fluorescence microscopy. This apparently simple method allows for quantifying CTC and was successfully used to detect CTC in peripheral blood of breast cancer patients.[24] Several new *in vivo* imaging procedures to detect cancer-associated biomarkers, although thus far limited for usage in animal models, have been developed for the visualization of rare cells, with great potential for future application also in humans. Intravital flow cytometry, for instance, noninvasively counts CTC *in vivo* as they flow through the peripheral vasculature. Here, multiphoton fluorescence imaging of superficial blood vessels follows i.v. injection of a tumor-specific fluorescent ligand to quantify flowing CTC. Using this approach, CTC could be detected and quantified in mice weeks before metastatic disease was detectable by other methods.[25] Another new device circumventing the problem of limited availability of blood volume for CTC analysis, which has already successfully been applied in mouse models, is *in vivo* photoacoustic (PA) flow cytometry (PAFC), which integrates *in vivo* multiplex targeting, magnetic enrichment, signal amplification, and multicolor recognition. Magnetic nanoparticles functionalized to target receptors commonly found in breast cancer cells, such as urokinase plasminogen activator receptor or the stem cell marker CD44, bind and capture CTC under a magnet. Magnetic capturing of CTC in the bloodstream of mice is followed by rapid PA detection. Gold-plated carbon nanotubes conjugated with folic acid are used as a second contrast agent for PA imaging to improve sensitivity and specificity. This device has the potential to detect CTC in blood and lymph flow, as well as to monitor therapies in real-time through the counting of circulating abnormal objects.[26]

Flow cytometry-based methods have also been used for CTC detection, but are generally hampered by the extremely rare number of CTC, and therefore have mainly been described for blood analysis from patients with overt metastases.[27] Improvements in multiparameter flow cytometry will enable effective CTC detection, with the potential to be a valuable tool for prognosis assessment in cancer patients.[28]

The recently presented "CTC-chip," a microfluid platform consisting of anti-EpCAM antibody-coated microposts capable of capturing CTC from unfractionated blood under precisely controlled laminar flow conditions, revealed positive events in almost all cancer patients, independent of the stage of the disease.[29] Using this device Maheswaran and colleagues demonstrated that CTC from lung cancer patients share common mutations in the EGFR gene with in the corresponding primary tumors.[30] Recent improvements of the CTC chip technology led to reduced numbers of CTC, which were more comparable with reports using other assays in comparable patient populations.[31] Large scale multi-center studies are now required to validate this promising technology. Another microfluidic device, equipped with a size-selective microcavity array for highly efficient and rapid detection of tumor cells from whole blood, was developed by Hosokawa and colleagues, however, the impact of this approach for the evaluation of patient samples has still to be elucidated.[32]

The MagSweeper, an automated immunomagnetic separation technology allowing further molecular characterization of CTC, was presented very recently by Talasaz.[33] With a specialized laser scanning cytometer (MAINTRAC^{TM} assay) CTC counts 2–3 log units higher than those obtained by the FDA-approved CellSearch method reported by Pachmann and colleagues in nearly 100% of breast cancer patients.[34] This CTC detection method also is based on EpCAM expression by CTC; however, careful validation studies are warranted to confirm specificity of this detection system, which results in extremely high counts of positive events (e.g., up to 10^5 per mL blood) that may not be tumor cells. Other automated fluorescence-scanning microscopic devices have been introduced, with promising results for evaluation of immunocytochemically stained blood samples enriched for rare cells by different approaches, but these techniques also need to be validated in large clinical studies.[35,36] Multichannel devices are of particular interest because they enable detection of several markers in parallel, e.g., in cells that have lost their characteristic epithelial markers in the course of epithelial–mesenchymal transition.

Furthermore, ultra-speed automated digital microscopy fiber-optic array scanning technology (FAST) and laser printing techniques allow ultra fast evaluation of images,[37] thus detecting CTC labeled by fluorescence-dye-conjugated antibodies mounted directly on a slide. Identification and differentiation of single tumor cells from peripheral blood by Raman spectroscopic label-free imaging, studying vibrational, rotational, and other low-frequency modes in a system, might become a useful tool to distinguish tumor cells from white blood cells. With the micro-Raman set up described by Neugebauer and colleagues, detailed biochemical information of individual cells, with a spatial resolution in the submicometer range, can be obtained.[38] This technique was already successfully used for discriminating between normal and diseased cells and for following processes involved in the differentiation of stem cells.[38] The newly developed microfluidic flow-through electroporation technique is still limited to mouse models and takes advantage of the different responses of tumor cells and blood cells to electroporation; it allows for the observation of electroporation in real time and therefore might be useful for analyzing CTC.[39]

Circulating cell-free DNA derived from tumor cells harbors detectable genetic aberrations and has the potential to serve as surrogate for CTC. Recent data showed that this cell-free DNA is significantly associated with the presence of CTC in blood or DTC in BM of prostate cancer patients.[40] There is also evidence for specific microRNA in peripheral blood being a new tool for monitoring CTC in cancer patients, as recently shown for patients with gastric cancer.[41]

The use of reverse transcriptase (RT)-PCR to detect epithelium-specific or rather organ-specific transcripts such as CK19, MUC-1, HER2, or mammaglobin has also been proven as a promising means to detect CTC/DTC.[42–45] A commercially available RT-PCR test called Adnatest Breast Cancer Detect analyzes tumor-associated mRNA for HER2, MUC1, or GA 733–2 as markers of CTC in blood from primary breast cancer patients.[46] Very recently, van der Auwera and colleagues reported a study that compared three techniques to detect CTC in blood samples from 76 patients with metastatic breast cancer (MBC) and from 20 healthy controls using the CellSearch CTC System, the AdnaTest Breast Cancer Select/Detect, and a previously developed real-time qRT-PCR assay for the detection of CK-19 and mammaglobin transcripts. The highest rate of CTC-positivity was observed using a combined qRT-PCR approach for CK-19 and mammaglobin, which is consistent with the conclusion that this is currently the most sensitive technique for detecting CTC.[47] On the other side, Helo and colleagues demonstrated that RT-PCR and CellSearch CTC results were strongly concordant and correlated in patients with localized prostate cancer and CRPC.[48] However, the main drawback of RT-PCR approaches is the lack of specificity resulting from false positive results due to "illegitimate" low-level epithelial- or tissue-related transcription in normal cells.[49] Moreover, heterogeneity in the expression of a particular target transcript may affect the analysis and expression of individual cells that cannot be validated. Nevertheless, several studies have provided evidence for clinical relevance of CTC detected by RT-PCR.[2,50]

Characterization of diagnostically and therapeutically relevant features of CTC/DTC

Further characterization of CTC is pivotal for insight into the complex biology of tumor cell spread, with important implications for defining therapeutic targets and eliminating MRD.

Detection of genomic aberrations

For DTC in bone marrow a striking genetic disparity between primary tumors was described by Klein and colleagues.[51,52] Results from earlier studies suggest that DTC in bone marrow might be genomically unstable and heterogeneous,[53] as well as capable of dissemination in a less progressed genomic state by acquiring genomic alterations typical for fully metastatic cells later.[54] Direct genetic analysis of single DTC from patients with esophageal cancer, by whole genome screening, identified gains in the HER2 encoding region as the most frequent amplification in DTC, and associated with a high risk of early death.[55]

Because of the high number of detectable CTC in patients with castration-resistant prostate cancer (CRPC), the majority of results concerning genetic aberrations published thus far are from CRPC patients. Genotyping using oligonucleotide array comparative genomic hybridization revealed copy number profiles in CTC from CRPC patients similar to those observed in paired tumor tissues.[56] By multicolor fluorescence in situ hybridization (FISH), homogeneity in ERG oncogene rearrangement status in CTC from CRPC patients was observed in contrast to significant heterogeneity of androgen receptor (AR) copy number gain and PTEN loss.[57] That the majority of CTC in hormone refractory prostate cancer are aneuploid was shown by Swennenhuis and colleagues, confirming that these cells are cancer cells. Furthermore, heterogeneous copy numbers of chromosomes 1, 7, 8, and 17 were observed.[58] In a considerable number of CTC samples from patients with CRPC, amplifications of the AR gene locus could be detected.[15,59] Very recently, mutations in the gene encoding AR were identified in CTC-enriched peripheral blood samples from CRPC patients by applying Transgenomic's

WAVE(R) denaturing HPLC technology followed by direct sequencing.[60]

Gene expression analysis

In DTC, heterogeneity with respect to the expression of growth factor receptors, adhesion molecules, proteases and their inducer and receptors, major histocompatibility complex antigens, signaling kinases, melanoma associated antigens (MAGE), or telomerase activity has been observed.[1,3,61–63] Most DTC and CTC were detected in a nonproliferative state, as revealed by Ki-67 immunostainings.[6,7] Expression of hypoxia-inducible factor-1alpha (HIF-1alpha), vascular endothelial growth factor (VEGF), and VEGF-receptor (VEGFR2), associated with angiogenesis and tumor progression, was shown in CTC and DTC of breast cancer patients.[64]

The epidermal growth factor receptor HER2, the expression of which in primary tumors is the basis for trastuzumab treatment decisions of breast cancer patients,[65] has gained particular interest. As Braun and colleagues demonstrated, HER2 overexpression on DTC in bone marrow is predictive for a poor clinical outcome of stage I–III breast cancer patients.[66] Vincent-Salomon and colleagues demonstrated that in the majority of cases, the HER2 status remained stable between DTC and the corresponding primary tumors.[67] However, most published studies suggest that there are discrepancies between the HER2 status in primary tumors and DTC in bone marrow[66,68] and CTC in blood (Fig. 1).[18,69–72]

Global gene expression profiles of CTC from patients with metastatic, breast cancer might be useful to distinguish normal donors from cancer patients.[73] TWIST1, a transcription factor pivotal for metastasis, by promoting epithelial–mesenchymal transition,[74] was part of the gene expression signature identified in EpCAM-enriched cells from bone marrow of breast cancer patients after chemotherapy, and its expression was associated with distant metastasis and local progression.[75]

Balic and colleagues and Alix-Panabieres and colleagues, who demonstrated a significant number of DTC from bone marrow of breast cancer patients with either CD44$^+$/CD24$^{-/low}$ or CK19$^+$/Muc-1$^-$ stem cell-like phenotypes, provided first hints for stem cell features of DTC in bone marrow.[21,76] With the AdnaTestTumorStemCell/TheAdnaTestEMT RT-PCT assay, Aktas and colleagues identified features characteristic of stem cells and of EMT in a major proportion of CTC from metastatic breast cancer patients.[77] A subpopulation of CTC with the putative stem cell phenotypes CD44$^+$/CD24$^{-/low}$ or ALDH1high/CD24$^{-/low}$ was recently reported in a subpopulation of patients with metastatic breast cancer, using triple-marker immunofluorescence microscopy.[78] In a subset of breast cancer stem cells with the potential to self-renewal, Notch seems to represent a genetic biomarker that is more frequently co-expressed with HER2 than associated with a HER2-negative phenotype.[79] Also indicative for a putative stem cell phenotype is the observed resistance of DTC in BM of cancer patients to systemic chemotherapy and their long term persistence.[80,81] In a recently published study, Gazzaniga and colleagues identified a putative drug-resistance profile of CTC with a predictive value for response to chemotherapy, independent of the tumor type and the stage of the disease; this provides relevance for the individualization of chemotherapy in cancer patients.[82]

Clinical relevance of CTC detection

The application of DTC and CTC analyses was mentioned for the first time in 2007 in the American Society of Oncology (ASCO) recommendations on tumor markers.[83] This was at least partly based on results of a meta-analysis published by Braun and colleagues including data of 4703 breast cancer patients, demonstrating that the presence of DTC in bone marrow was not only predictive of the development of skeletal metastases but also predicted the development of metastases in other organs.[84] Although most results on the clinical relevance of DTC/CTC have been obtained for patients with breast cancer, there is increasing evidence for a pivotal role of MRD analysis also in patients with other solid tumors.[2,50]

CTC/DTC are able to survive chemotherapy and hormonal therapy[6,85] as well as to persist in bone marrow over many years post-surgery, which is probably associated with an increased risk of late metastatic relapse.[80,81,86] As evidenced by a European pooled analysis involving 696 breast cancer patients, persistence of DTC in 16% of breast cancer patients was an independent prognostic factor for subsequent reduced breast cancer survival.[87] The prognostic relevance of DTC detection in stage I to III breast cancer patients was shown recently,[88] and

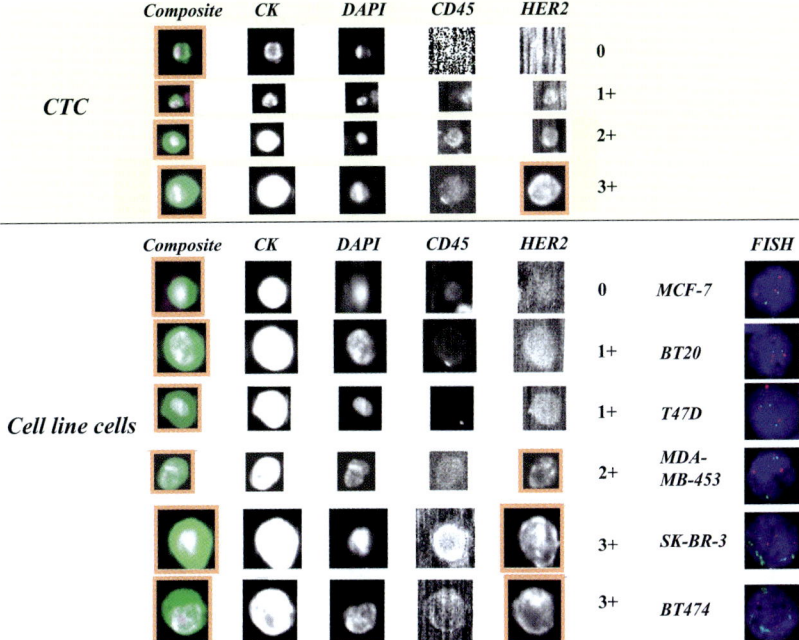

Figure 1. Determination of the HER2 status of CTC with the CellSearch system. CTC are cytokeratin (CK)-, and DAPI (4′,6-diamidin-2′-phenylindol-dihydrochlorid)-positive and CD45-negative. HER2 expression of CTC and breast cancer cell line cells spiked into blood was determined using a FITC (fluorescein isothiocyanate)-labeled anti HER2 antibody (tumor-phenotyping reagent HER-2/neu, Veridex, Raritan, NJ, USA) in the CellSearch system. Intensities of HER2-specific immunofluorescence of CTC were categorized into negative (0), weak (1+), moderate (2+), and strong (3+) by comparing the results for CTC with those obtained with cell line cells. FISH, lower right panel: HER2 gene amplification of breast cancer cell line cells was determined by FISH (fluorescence *in situ* hybridization, green signals: HER2; red signals: centromer 17).

the presence of DTC in bone marrow was associated with a different pattern of locoregional cancer cell dissemination, obviously being influencing locoregional recurrence-free survival as well.[89]

To implement screenings for MRD into clinical studies, besides other important requirements, repeated sample collection must be feasible. In this context, sequential peripheral blood analyses are more convenient than bone marrow analyses. However, there is still a limited number of studies that have directly compared bone marrow and blood analyses in the same patients.[6,90,91] Only studies on larger cohorts of patients may help to conclusively clarify whether blood analyses have the capacity to replace the bone marrow test.

Encouraging results concerning an association between CTC detection and metastatic progression in patients with metastatic breast, prostate, and colorectal cancer have been recently published.[11,13,15,92–94] Results by Hayes and colleagues indicated that CTC in peripheral blood of metastatic

breast cancer patients at any time during therapy directly reflect the patient's response, or lack of response, respectively, to therapy[12] and are therefore superior or additive to conventional imaging methods.[13,95,96] Nevertheless, the recent ASCO guidelines do not recommend the use of the FDA-cleared CellSearch assay in patients with metastatic breast cancer until further validation confirms the clinical value of this test.[83] The randomized trial SWOG S0500 led by the Southwest Oncology group (www.cancer.gov/clinicaltrials/SWOG-S0500, last modified 10/23/2008[97]), expecting to enroll 500 patients with metastatic breast cancer, prospectively addresses the clinical utility of CTC measurements in metastatic breast cancer patients.

A challenging task for new techniques intended to analyze CTC/DTC is to enable monitoring MRD in patients with nonmetastatic cancer. Recently, promising results derived from patients with nonmetastatic breast cancer enrolled in neoadjuvant treatment studies. The presence of CTC after a short follow-up time of 18 months was an independent prognostic factor for reduced metastasis-free survival in a phase II trial (REMAGUS 02) in which 118 patients with large operable or locally advanced breast cancer before and after neoadjuvant chemotherapy were monitored for CTC.[98] After an extension of the median follow-up to 36 months, CTC detection before chemotherapy became an independent prognostic factor for both distant metastasis-free survival and overall survival.[99] In this neoadjuvant-treated patient cohort, there was no significant correlation between neoadjuvant use and response of the primary tumor to chemotherapy, which is the current standard method to assess therapeutic efficacy in neoadjuvant therapies. Thus, measuring changes in CTC counts may provide additional information on the response of an individual patient. Follow up analyses of two German trials using the CellSearch technology—the GEPARQuattro trial on neoadjuvant chemotherapy and trastuzumab treatment, and the SUCCESS trial on adjuvant chemotherapy—are still ongoing and will show whether the observed decreases in CTC rates are associated with an improved survival rate.[72,100] As recently described by Xenidis and colleagues, patients with detectable CK19 mRNA post chemotherapy had a significantly reduced overall and disease-free survival.[45] Additional information of the expression of important target molecules on CTC, such as HER2 and EGFR might be helpful for future stratification and monitoring of targeted therapies such as trastuzumab or lapatinib.

Conclusions and future directions

A considerable number of rare cell detection techniques have been developed during the last years that are being continuously improved by several working groups. These techniques help detect DTC in bone marrow and of CTC in blood of cancer patients years before the occurrence of distant overt metastases. Nevertheless, analysis of DTC/CTC is still not part of the routine tumor staging in clinical practice. This is mainly due to the low number of these cells detectable with the currently available methods, limiting their value as a so-called "liquid biopsy," especially in patients with early stage tumors. Therefore, new innovative approaches urgently have to be evaluated for reproducibility, sensitivity, and specificity in order to become applicable for clinical practice. Information about CTC/DTC

status may be used to assess prognosis of cancer patients and to stratify the patients at risk to systemic therapies aimed to prevent recurrences and metastatic relapses. Furthermore, CTC/DTC measurements within clinical trials might serve as an important biomarker for real-time monitoring of the efficacy of systemic therapies in individual cancer patients, and might thereby support accelerating drug development and defining subpopulations of patients with the highest treatment benefit. Moreover, CTC/DTC analysis for downstream components within signal transducing pathways, which influence new targeted therapies (e.g., K-ras mutations in EGFR-targeted therapies or PI3K mutations in HER2-targeted therapies), might provide new insights into the complex mechanisms of drug resistance.

Conflicts of interest

The authors declare no conflicts of interest.

References

1. Pantel, K., R.H. Brakenhoff & B. Brandt. 2008. Detection, clinical relevance and specific biological properties of disseminating tumour cells. *Nat. Rev. Cancer* **8:** 329–340.
2. Pantel, K., C. Alix-Panabieres & S. Riethdorf. 2009. Cancer micrometastases. *Nat. Rev. Clin. Oncol.* **6:** 339–351.
3. Pantel, K. & R.H. Brakenhoff. 2004. Dissecting the metastatic cascade. *Nat. Rev. Cancer* **4:** 448–456.
4. Kim, M.Y. *et al.* 2009. Tumor self-seeding by circulating cancer cells. *Cell* **139:** 1315–1326.
5. Cristofanilli, M. & S. Braun. Circulating tumor cells revisited. *JAMA* **303:** 1092–1093.
6. Muller, V. *et al.* 2005. Circulating tumor cells in breast cancer: correlation to bone marrow micrometastases, heterogeneous response to systemic therapy and low proliferative activity. *Clin. Cancer Res.* **11:** 3678–3685.
7. Pantel, K. *et al.* 1993. Differential expression of proliferation-associated molecules in individual micrometastatic carcinoma cells. *J. Natl. Cancer Inst.* **85:** 1419–1424.
8. Alix-Panabieres, C., S. Riethdorf & K. Pantel. 2008. Circulating tumor cells and bone marrow micrometastasis. *Clin. Cancer Res.* **14:** 5013–5021.
9. Lacroix, M. 2006. Significance, detection and markers of disseminated breast cancer cells. *Endocr. Relat. Cancer* **13:** 1033–1067.
10. Fehm, T. *et al.* 2006. A concept for the standardized detection of disseminated tumor cells in bone marrow from patients with primary breast cancer and its clinical implementation. *Cancer* **107:** 885–892.
11. Cristofanilli, M. *et al.* 2004. Circulating tumor cells, disease progression, and survival in metastatic breast cancer. *N. Engl. J. Med.* **351:** 781–791.

12. Hayes, D.F. *et al.* 2006. Circulating tumor cells at each follow-up time point during therapy of metastatic breast cancer patients predict progression-free and overall survival. *Clin. Cancer Res.* **12:** 4218–4224.

13. Cohen, S.J. *et al.* 2008. Relationship of circulating tumor cells to tumor response, progression-free survival, and overall survival in patients with metastatic colorectal cancer. *J. Clin. Oncol.* **26:** 3213–3221.

14. Riethdorf, S. *et al.* 2007. Detection of circulating tumor cells in peripheral blood of patients with metastatic breast cancer: a validation study of the CellSearch system. *Clin. Cancer Res.* **13:** 920–928.

15. Shaffer, D.R. *et al.* 2007. Circulating tumor cell analysis in patients with progressive castration-resistant prostate cancer. *Clin. Cancer Res.* **13:** 2023–2029.

16. Sieuwerts, A.M. *et al.* 2009. Anti-epithelial cell adhesion molecule antibodies and the detection of circulating normal-like breast tumor cells. *J. Natl. Cancer Inst.* **101:** 61–66.

17. Lalmahomed, Z.S. *et al.* 2010. Circulating tumor cells and sample size: the more, the better. *J. Clin. Oncol.* **28:** e288–e289; author reply e290.

18. Flores, L.M. *et al.* 2010. Improving the yield of circulating tumour cells facilitates molecular characterisation and recognition of discordant HER2 amplification in breast cancer. *Br. J. Cancer* **102:** 1495–1502.

19. Mostert, B. *et al.* 2010. Detection of circulating tumor cells in breast cancer may improve through enrichment with anti-CD146. *Breast Cancer Res. Treat.* Epub ahead of print.

20. Coumans, F.A., C.J. Doggen, G. Attard, *et al.* 2010. All circulating EpCAM+CK+CD45- objects predict overall survival in castration-resistant prostate cancer. *Ann. Oncol.* **21:** 1851–1857.

21. Alix-Panabieres, C. *et al.* 2007. Detection and characterization of putative metastatic precursor cells in cancer patients. *Clin. Chem.* **53:** 537–539.

22. Alix-Panabieres, C. *et al.* 2009. Full length cytokeratin-19 is released by human tumor cells: a potential role in metastatic progression of breast cancer. *Breast Cancer Res.* **11:** R39.

23. Lu, J. *et al.* 2010. Isolation of circulating epithelial and tumor progenitor cells with an invasive phenotype from breast cancer patients. *Int. J. Cancer* **126:** 669–683.

24. Kojima, T. *et al.* 2009. A simple biological imaging system for detecting viable human circulating tumor cells. *J. Clin. Invest.* **119:** 3172–3181.

25. He, W., H. Wang, L.C. Hartmann, *et al.* 2007. in vivo quantitation of rare circulating tumor cells by multiphoton intravital flow cytometry. *Proc. Natl. Acad. Sci. USA* **104:** 11760–11765.

26. Galanzha, E.I. *et al.* 2009. in vivo magnetic enrichment and multiplex photoacoustic detection of circulating tumour cells. *Nat. Nanotechnol.* **4:** 855–860.

27. Garcia, J.A. *et al.* 2007. Evaluation and significance of circulating epithelial cells in patients with hormone-refractory prostate cancer. *BJU Int.* **99:** 519–524.

28. Hu, Y. *et al.* 2010. Detection of circulating tumor cells in breast cancer patients utilizing multiparameter flow cytometry and assessment of the prognosis of patients in different CTCs levels. *Cytometry A* **77:** 213–219.

29. Nagrath, S. *et al.* 2007. Isolation of rare circulating tumour cells in cancer patients by microchip technology. *Nature* **450:** 1235–1239.

30. Maheswaran, S. *et al.* 2008. Detection of mutations in EGFR in circulating lung-cancer cells. *N. Engl. J. Med.* **359:** 366–377.

31. Stott, S.L. *et al.* 2010. Isolation and characterization of circulating tumor cells from patients with localized and metastatic prostate cancer. *Sci. Trans. Med.* **2:** 25ra23.

32. Hosokawa, M. *et al.* 2010. Size-Selective Microcavity Array for Rapid and Efficient Detection of Circulating Tumor Cells. *Anal. Chem.* **82:** 6629–6635.

33. Talasaz, A.H. *et al.* 2009. Isolating highly enriched populations of circulating epithelial cells and other rare cells from blood using a magnetic sweeper device. *Proc. Natl. Acad. Sci. USA* **106:** 3970–3975.

34. Pachmann, K. *et al.* 2005. Standardized quantification of circulating peripheral tumor cells from lung and breast cancer. *Clin. Chem. Lab. Med.* **43:** 617–627.

35. Deng, G. *et al.* 2008. Enrichment with anti-cytokeratin alone or combined with anti-EpCAM antibodies significantly increases the sensitivity for circulating tumor cell detection in metastatic breast cancer patients. *Breast Cancer Res.* **10:** R69.

36. Ntouroupi, T.G. *et al.* 2008. Detection of circulating tumour cells in peripheral blood with an automated scanning fluorescence microscope. *Br. J. Cancer* **99:** 789–795.

37. Hsieh, H.B. *et al.* 2006. High speed detection of circulating tumor cells. *Biosens. Bioelectron.* **21:** 1893–1899.

38. Neugebauer, U., J.H. Clement, T. Bocklitz, *et al.* 2010. Identification and differentiation of single cells from peripheral blood by Raman spectroscopic imaging. *J. Biophotonic.* **3:** 579–587.

39. Bao, N., T.T. Le, J.X. Cheng & C. Lu. 2010. Microfluidic electroporation of tumor and blood cells: observation of nucleus expansion and implications on selective analysis and purging of circulating tumor cells. *Integr. Biol. (Camb.)* **2:** 113–120.

40. Schwarzenbach, H. *et al.* 2009. Cell-free tumor DNA in blood plasma as a marker for circulating tumor cells in prostate cancer. *Clin. Cancer Res.* **15:** 1032–1038.

41. Zhou, H. *et al.* 2010. Detection of circulating tumor cells in peripheral blood from patients with gastric cancer using microRNA as a marker. *J. Mol. Med.* **88:** 709–717.

42. Berois, N. *et al.* 2000. Molecular detection of cancer cells in bone marrow and peripheral blood of patients with operable breast cancer. Comparison of CK19, MUC1 and CEA using RT-PCR. *Eur. J. Cancer* **36:** 717–723.

43. Bossolasco, P. *et al.* 2002. Detection of micrometastatic cells in breast cancer by RT-pCR for the mammaglobin gene. *Cancer Detect. Prev.* **26:** 60–63.

44. Ignatiadis, M. *et al.* 2008. Prognostic Value of the Molecular Detection of Circulating Tumor Cells Using a Multimarker Reverse Transcription-PCR Assay for Cytokeratin 19, Mammaglobin A, and HER2 in Early Breast Cancer. *Clin. Cancer Res.* **14:** 2593–2600.

45. Xenidis, N. *et al.* 2009. Cytokeratin-19 mRNA-positive circulating tumor cells after adjuvant chemotherapy in

patients with early breast cancer. *J. Clin. Oncol.* **27:** 2177–2184.

46. Fehm, T. *et al.* 2009. Detection and characterization of circulating tumor cells in blood of primary breast cancer patients by RT-PCR and comparison to status of bone marrow disseminated cells. *Breast Cancer Res.* **11:** R59.

47. Van Der Auwera, I. *et al.* (2010. Circulating tumour cell detection: a direct comparison between the CellSearch System, the AdnaTest and CK-19/mammaglobin RT-PCR in patients with metastatic breast cancer. *Br. J. Cancer* **102:** 276–284.

48. Helo, P. *et al.* 2009. Circulating prostate tumor cells detected by reverse transcription-PCR in men with localized or castration-refractory prostate cancer: concordance with CellSearch assay and association with bone metastases and with survival. *Clin. Chem.* **55:** 765–773.

49. Ballestrero, A. *et al.* 2005. Effect of different cytokines on mammaglobin and maspin gene expression in normal leukocytes: possible relevance to the assays for the detection of micrometastatic breast cancer. *Br. J. Cancer* **92:** 1948–1952.

50. Riethdorf, S., H. Wikman & K. Pantel. 2008. Review: biological relevance of disseminated tumor cells in cancer patients. *Int. J. Cancer* **123:** 1991–2006.

51. Klein, C.A. & N.H. Stoecklein. 2009. Lessons from an aggressive cancer: evolutionary dynamics in esophageal carcinoma. *Cancer Res.* **69:** 5285–5288.

52. Stoecklein, N.H. & C.A. Klein. 2010. Genetic disparity between primary tumours, disseminated tumour cells, and manifest metastasis. *Int. J. Cancer* **126:** 589–598.

53. Klein, C.A. *et al.* 2002. Genetic heterogeneity of single disseminated tumour cells in minimal residual cancer. *Lancet* **360:** 683–689.

54. Schmidt-Kittler, O. *et al.* 2003. From latent disseminated cells to overt metastasis: genetic analysis of systemic breast cancer progression. *Proc. Natl. Acad. Sci. USA* **100:** 7737–7742.

55. Stoecklein, N.H. *et al.* 2008. Direct genetic analysis of single disseminated cancer cells for prediction of outcome and therapy selection in esophageal cancer. *Cancer Cell.* **13:** 441–453.

56. Paris, P.L. *et al.* 2009. Functional phenotyping and genotyping of circulating tumor cells from patients with castration resistant prostate cancer. *Cancer Lett.* **277:** 164–173.

57. Attard, G. *et al.* 2009. Characterization of ERG, AR and PTEN gene status in circulating tumor cells from patients with castration-resistant prostate cancer. *Cancer Res.* **69:** 2912–2918.

58. Swennenhuis, J.F., A.G. Tibbe, R. Levink, *et al.* 2009. Characterization of circulating tumor cells by fluorescence in situ hybridization. Cytometry A **75:** 520–527.

59. Leversha, M.A. *et al.* 2009. Fluorescence in situ hybridization analysis of circulating tumor cells in metastatic prostate cancer. *Clin. Cancer Res.* **15:** 2091–2097.

60. Jiang, Y., J.F. Palma, D.B. Agus, *et al.* 2010. Detection of Androgen Receptor Mutations in Circulating Tumor Cells in Castration-Resistant Prostate Cancer. *Clin. Chem.* **56:** 7492–7495.

61. Pantel, K. *et al.* 1991. Frequent down-regulation of major histocompatibility class I antigen expression on individual micrometastatic carcinoma cells. *Cancer Res.* **51:** 4712–4715.

62. Klein, C.A. *et al.* 2002. Combined transcriptome and genome analysis of single micrometastatic cells. *Nat. Biotechnol.* **20:** 387–392.

63. Pierga, J.Y. *et al.* 2005. Real-time quantitative PCR determination of urokinase-type plasminogen activator receptor (uPAR) expression of isolated micrometastatic cells from bone marrow of breast cancer patients. *Int. J. Cancer* **114:** 291–298.

64. Kallergi, G. *et al.* 2009. Hypoxia-inducible factor-1alpha and vascular endothelial growth factor expression in circulating tumor cells of breast cancer patients. *Breast Cancer Res.* **11:** R84.

65. Piccart-Gebhart, M.J. *et al.* 2005. Trastuzumab after adjuvant chemotherapy in HER2-positive breast cancer. *N. Engl. J. Med.* **353:** 1659–1672.

66. Braun, S. *et al.* 2001. ErbB2 overexpression on occult metastatic cells in bone marrow predicts poor clinical outcome of stage I-III breast cancer patients. *Cancer Res.* **61:** 1890–1895.

67. Vincent-Salomon, A. *et al.* 2007. HER2 status of bone marrow micrometastasis and their corresponding primary tumours in a pilot study of 27 cases: a possible tool for anti-HER2 therapy management? *Br. J. Cancer* **96:** 654–659.

68. Solomayer, E.F. *et al.* 2006. Comparison of HER2 status between primary tumor and disseminated tumor cells in primary breast cancer patients. *Breast Cancer Res. Treat.* **98:** 179–184.

69. Meng, S. *et al.* 2004. HER-2 gene amplification can be acquired as breast cancer progresses. *Proc. Natl. Acad. Sci. USA* **101:** 9393–9398.

70. Wulfing, P. *et al.* 2006. HER2-positive circulating tumor cells indicate poor clinical outcome in stage I to III breast cancer patients. *Clin. Cancer Res.* **12:** 1715–1720.

71. Krawczyk, N. *et al.* 2009. HER2 status on persistent disseminated tumor cells after adjuvant therapy may differ from initial HER2 status on primary tumor. *Anticancer. Res.* **29:** 4019–4024.

72. Riethdorf, S. *et al.* 2010. Detection and HER2 expression of circulating tumor cells: prospective monitoring in breast cancer patients treated in the neoadjuvant GeparQuattro trial. *Clin. Cancer Res.* **16:** 2634–2645.

73. Smirnov, D.A. *et al.* 2005. Global gene expression profiling of circulating tumor cells. *Cancer Res.* **65:** 4993–4997.

74. Rosivatz, E. *et al.* 2002. Differential expression of the epithelial-mesenchymal transition regulators snail, SIP1, and twist in gastric cancer. *Am. J. Pathol.* **161:** 1881–1891.

75. Watson, M.A. *et al.* 2007. Isolation and molecular profiling of bone marrow micrometastases identifies TWIST1 as a marker of early tumor relapse in breast cancer patients. *Clin. Cancer Res.* **13:** 5001–5009.

76. Balic, M. *et al.* 2006. Most early disseminated cancer cells detected in bone marrow of breast cancer patients have a putative breast cancer stem cell phenotype. *Clin. Cancer Res.* **12:** 5615–5621.

77. Aktas, B. *et al.* 2009. Stem cell and epithelial-mesenchymal transition markers are frequently overexpressed in circulating tumor cells of metastatic breast cancer patients. *Breast Cancer Res.* **11,** R46.

78. Theodoropoulos, P.A. *et al.* 2010. Circulating tumor cells with a putative stem cell phenotype in peripheral blood of patients with breast cancer. *Cancer Lett.* **288:** 99–106.

79. Reuben, J.M. *et al.* 2010. Circulating tumor cells and biomarkers: implications for personalized targeted treatments for metastatic breast cancer. *Breast J.* **16:** 327–330.

80. Wiedswang, G. *et al.* 2004. Isolated tumor cells in bone marrow three years after diagnosis in disease-free breast cancer patients predict unfavorable clinical outcome. *Clin. Cancer Res.* **10:** 5342–5348.

81. Janni, W. *et al.* 2005. The persistence of isolated tumor cells in bone marrow from patients with breast carcinoma predicts an increased risk for recurrence. *Cancer* **103:** 884–891.

82. Gazzaniga, P. *et al.* 2010. Chemosensitivity profile assay of circulating cancer cells: prognostic and predictive value in epithelial tumors. *Int. J. Cancer* **126:** 2437–2447.

83. Harris, L. *et al.* 2007. American Society of Clinical Oncology 2007 update of recommendations for the use of tumor markers in breast cancer. *J. Clin. Oncol.* **25:** 5287–5312.

84. Braun, S. *et al.* 2005. A pooled analysis of bone marrow micrometastasis in breast cancer. *N. Engl. J. Med.* **353:** 793–802.

85. Braun, S. *et al.* 2000. Lack of effect of adjuvant chemotherapy on the elimination of single dormant tumor cells in bone marrow of high-risk breast cancer patients. *J. Clin. Oncol.* **18:** 80–86.

86. Slade, M.J. *et al.* 2005. Persistence of bone marrow micrometastases in patients receiving adjuvant therapy for breast cancer: results at 4 years. *Int. J. Cancer* **114:** 94–100.

87. Naume, B. *et al.* 2008. Persistence of isolated tumor cells in the bone marrow of breast cancer patients predicts increased risk for relapse—a European pooled analysis. *SABCS 2008* **#304.**

88. Bidard, F.C. *et al.* 2008. Disseminated tumor cells of breast cancer patients: a strong prognostic factor for distant and local relapse. *Clin. Cancer Res.* **14:** 3306–3311.

89. Bidard, F.C. *et al.* 2009. Disseminated tumor cells and the risk of locoregional recurrence in nonmetastatic breast cancer. *Ann. Oncol.* **20:** 1836–1841.

90. Wiedswang, G. *et al.* 2006. Comparison of the clinical significance of occult tumor cells in blood and bone marrow in breast cancer. *Int. J. Cancer* **118:** 2013–2019.

91. Bidard, F.C. *et al.* 2008. Prognosis of women with stage IV breast cancer depends on detection of circulating tumor cells rather than disseminated tumor cells. *Ann. Oncol.* **19:** 496–500.

92. de Bono, J.S. *et al.* 2007. Potential applications for circulating tumor cells expressing the insulin-like growth factor-I receptor. *Clin. Cancer Res.* **13:** 3611–3616.

93. de Bono, J.S. *et al.* 2008. Circulating tumor cells predict survival benefit from treatment in metastatic castration-resistant prostate cancer. *Clin Cancer Res* **14:** 6302–6309.

94. Danila, D.C. *et al.* 2007. Circulating tumor cell number and prognosis in progressive castration-resistant prostate cancer. *Clin. Cancer. Res.* **13:** 7053–7058.

95. Budd, G.T. *et al.* 2006. Circulating tumor cells versus imaging–predicting overall survival in metastatic breast cancer. *Clin. Cancer Res.* **12:** 6403–6409.

96. De Giorgi, U. *et al.* 2009. Circulating tumor cells and [18F]fluorodeoxyglucose positron emission tomography/computed tomography for outcome prediction in metastatic breast cancer. *J. Clin. Oncol.* **27:** 3303–3311.

97. Treatment decision making based on blood levels of tumor cells in women with metastatic breast cancer receiving chemotherapy. SWOG-S0500. Available at: www.cancer.gov/clinicaltrials.

98. Pierga, J.Y. *et al.* 2008. Circulating tumor cell detection predicts early metastatic relapse after neoadjuvant chemotherapy in large operable and locally advanced breast cancer in a phase II randomized trial. *Clin. Cancer Res.* **14:** 7004–7010.

99. Bidard, F.C. *et al.* 2010. Single circulating tumor cell detection and overall survival in nonmetastatic breast cancer. *Ann. Oncol.* **21:** 729–733

100. Rack, B.K. *et al.* 2010. Use of circulating tumor cells (CTC) in peripheral blood of breast cancer patients before and after adjuvant chemotherapy to predict risk for relapse: the SUCCESS trial. *J. Clin. Oncol.* **28:** abstract 1003.

Ann. N.Y. Acad. Sci. ISSN 0077-8923

ANNALS OF THE NEW YORK ACADEMY OF SCIENCES
Issue: *Toward Personalized Medicine for Cancer*

Breast cancer genomics: normal tissue and cancer markers

Michèl Schummer,[1] David Beatty,[1,2] and Nicole Urban[1]

[1]Molecular Diagnostics Program, Fred Hutchinson Cancer Research Center, Seattle, Washington. [2]Swedish Cancer Institute, Seattle, Washington

Address for correspondence: Michèl Schummer, Fred Hutchinson Cancer Research Center, 1100 Fairview Ave N, Mail Stop M2-B230, Seattle, WA 98109. mschumme@fhcrc.org

Mammography is a powerful screening tool for early detection of breast cancer, but it has limitations in terms of both specificity and sensitivity. Imaging tools such as MRI that complement mammography are too costly to serve as first-line screens. Recently, progress has been made on blood markers, particularly microRNAs and proteins. There are new methods for protein marker discovery directly in blood, but they are limited in the number of patients that can be examined. An alternative is to discover markers as transcripts in tissues, followed by development of blood protein tests for those that perform best. To identify genes that are overexpressed in malignancy it is paramount to include normal control tissues from healthy individuals. Here we report the identification of potential breast cancer markers, including some that are overexpressed in aggressive disease.

Keywords: normal breast tissue; cancer environment, aggressive breast cancer; early detection

Introduction

Breast cancer is the most common cancer diagnosed in women and the second most common cause of death from cancer among women in the United States.[1] A breast cancer is treated most effectively when the malignancy has not yet spread to other organs, that is, in its early stages.[1] The most common method for early detection of breast cancer is the use of mammography screening. Its introduction to the general population was associated with a progressive reduction of the mortality rate for breast cancer during the last two decades.[2] Its success is due to both mammography's ability to detect earlier forms of cancer and the concomitant development of better treatment options for breast cancer.

During the uptake of mammography, from 1980 to 1987, incidence rates of smaller invasive breast cancer ($\leq$2.0 cm) more than doubled, whereas rates of larger tumors (3.0 cm or more) decreased 27%.[2] Similarly, the incidence of noninvasive ductal carcinoma *in situ* (DCIS), a precursor of invasive breast cancer, rose from 1.87 per 100,000 in 1975 to 32.5 in 2004.[3] Ever since, mammography-detected DCIS

incidence has stabilized[1] at about 20% of breast cancers detected.[4]

Mammography is probably the best tool for screening a general population, but it is far from perfect. Of 100 women with breast cancer, screening mammography will miss about 10. This number varies with patient age[5,6] (higher in younger women), breast density[7–9] (higher in dense breasts) and infrastructure.[10] Although misses do not lead to direct harm to a woman, they provide her with the illusion of certainty of being disease-free. Such an illusion may at worst make women less attentive to physical symptoms of breast cancer.[11]

More frequently, a mammogram is positive when the patient has no malignancy. Reported false positive rates vary between countries and hospitals but are around 5%.[12,13] Applying the false-positive rate to the breast cancer cases diagnosed in the US in 2009 (123 per 100,000), to detect one woman's breast cancer with a screening mammogram, 20–50 women are falsely diagnosed every year. Interestingly, because the false-positive mammograms are cumulative and an average woman has more than one mammogram in her life, the odds for a false

doi: 10.1111/j.1749-6632.2010.05803.x

positive result rise over a patient's lifetime to as much as 43%.[12] In a 10-year retroactive study involving 2,400 patients, one third of screened women had an abnormal test result that required additional evaluation when no breast cancer was present.[14] The same study found that for every 100 dollars spent for screening, an additional 33 dollars was spent to evaluate the false positive results.[14]

In 1997, the Malmö Mammographic Screening Program showed that for every two breast cancer deaths prevented, one clinically insignificant cancer was diagnosed; for each breast cancer death prevented, 63 cancer-free women had been called back for further examinations; and for every 20 lives saved, one radiation-induced breast cancer death may have occurred. Recommendations for screening must therefore weigh mortality benefits against these negative effects.[15]

Although mammographic screening likely reduces breast cancer mortality,[16] it also leads to overdiagnosis and, resulting from it, overtreatment. Thus, in some circumstances, screening does more harm than good.

Alternatives to mammography

There is ample potential for an alternative screening method to complement mammography, thus reducing its false positive and false negative results. The method would need to be no more invasive than mammography, which makes biopsy not an option.

MRI can improve early cancer detection in high-risk women when used in conjunction with mammography.[17] It is recommended as a first-line screen for high-risk women[18] and for detecting cancer in a contralateral (opposite) breast.[19] Despite the fact that MRI is more expensive and less specific than mammography, it is more sensitive than mammography and is emerging as an important tool in the detection, diagnosis and staging of breast cancer.[20]

MicroRNAs are a new class of markers that can be measured directly in the blood. In a small study they were found to discriminate between cases and controls, even in early stages.[21] This area of research holds a lot of promise. There is even the rare examination of miRNA expression in male breast cancer.[22] MicroRNA markers thus have the same potential as traditional blood markers to complement mammography.

Although blood markers have been used for monitoring of breast cancer[23,24] or diagnosis of metastatic disease,[24] there is currently no blood marker that is used for early detection in the context of breast cancer screening.

Marker discovery in blood

Discovery of a marker for detection of cancer requires the comparison of healthy to diseased patient samples. For such comparisons to have meaningful results, the number of samples (patients and controls) need to be sufficiently high to allow for statistical analysis. Another important criterion is the number of analytes used in a study. In most cases these will be proteins, but lipids,[25–27] circulating tumor cells,[28,29] autoantibodies,[25,30–33] and microRNAs[21,34,35] have been reported as well. The larger the number of analytes in a study, the larger the sample needed to compensate for multiple comparisons and to minimize false discovery.

Finally, newly discovered markers need to be validated in larger, independent, and well-defined populations. Our experience has shown that the majority of serum markers that discriminate cancer cases from controls in studies with small samples sizes perform poorly in well-defined populations with 1,000 samples or more. This is often due to overfitting in the small studies, biased patient samples (e.g., cases and controls come from different hospitals), or inadequate annotation of the samples.

To discover markers that can identify women with cancer using blood samples, the most straightforward approach would be the direct comparison of serum or plasma from breast cancer patients to that of healthy controls. The most common method of protein discovery in blood is 2D gel analysis[36–38] but mass spectrometry is slowly gaining ground.[39,40] Unfortunately, for breast cancer the latter has resulted in peak patterns rather than proteins. Validation studies require proteins to be measured by ELISA because mass spectrometry is currently not suited for the analysis of a large number of patient samples. Thus, mass spectrometry is currently not a contender in the field for markers to complement mammography.

Using bead-based ELISAs, Jesneck and colleagues determined serum levels of 100 proteins in 53 breast cancer cases, 49 women with benign breast lesions, and 68 healthy controls. They found that three of the proteins discriminated between cancer cases and healthy controls, but they were also elevated in the benign cases compared to the controls, suggesting that these proteins play a role in inflammatory response to a lesion rather than in malignancy.[41] Our own data are more encouraging, particularly when focusing on subpopulations, such as women with dense breasts and women with aggressive cancers. We are hopeful that as the field evolves the promise of blood markers will be realized.

Marker discovery in tissue

Protein discovery in the blood has not yet yielded the desired results. It is however possible to make a detour through the tissue transcriptome to achieve the same goal. Compared to proteins, transcripts have several advantages: for discovery, there are well-established cost effective methods, and for expression validation, the methods can easily be ramped up to thousands of transcripts in thousands of samples. Although cancer-related transcripts can be found in circulating tumor cells,[28] the vast majority of all transcript-based experiments were performed in tissue. Many potential transcript-based cancer markers are reported in the literature but few of them have been validated either as transcripts in tissue or as protein in tissue. We know that there is significant correlation between transcript and protein expression in mammalian tissue or cells in cancers,[42,43] porcine tissues,[44] and cell lines,[45–47] but very little is known about the correlation of a tissue transcript with its cognate blood protein.

Our own marker discovery in ovarian cancer resulted in transcripts with overexpression in cancer tissues compared to normal tissues,[48] and the proteins they code for were later proven to be overexpressed in cancer sera compared to those from healthy individuals.[49–52] It should be noted however that correlation of overexpression of a marker (transcript in tissue and protein in blood) was observed on the level of a population rather than the individual.

The markers in our ovarian studies all coded for proteins that localized to the outside of the cell, either secreted or expressed in the extracellular matrix. We therefore postulate that, given a transcript that is (a) differentially expressed between cancer tissue and normal tissue from healthy individuals and (b) coding for a protein localized outside of the cell, the protein is likely to be differentially expressed in the blood.

Marker discovery through comparison of healthy to cancerous breast tissue

Over the last decade a large number of potential breast cancer markers have been discovered. The majority of them stem from experiments surrounding metastatic cancer or cancer-causing mechanisms using cell lines and mouse models. Publications using normal breast tissues from healthy donors are scarce.[53–56]

We recently reported[56] the results from a transcript-profiling study in breast cancer tissues and normal breast tissues from women without cancer in which we performed quantitative real-time PCR on two sets of transcripts: (1) 134 transcripts were identified by mining of publicly available expression data for genes with expression in breast cancer but not in normal tissues, coding for proteins with extracellular localization and low expression in organs with high cardiac output; and (2) 606 transcripts came precompiled on a commercial PCR platform (Cancer Pathways OpenArray, Life Technologies) stemming largely from the general cancer literature. We extracted RNA from 93 tissues (24 invasive cancers, 38 ipsilateral normal breast tissue, 3 contralateral normal breast tissue, 28 tissues from breast reduction surgery) from 64 women and performed unsupervised cluster analysis to identify among sets (a) and (b) those transcripts that discriminated between breast cancer tissues and normal breast tissues. For the genes found through mining, this resulted in 67 differentially expressed transcripts, 50% of them overexpressed in the cancer tissues. The Cancer Pathways OpenArray experiment resulted in 112 differentially expressed transcripts, 89% of them underexpressed in the breast cancer tissues. We assume that this discrepancy lies in the selection process for each set: the Cancer Pathways genes had been selected based on general cancer literature that includes a large number of within-cancer and cell line experiments. Hence, the set contains many transcripts coding for intracellular and regulatory proteins. Our data mining on the other hand focused on differences between breast cancer and normal breast tissue and on extracellular expression.

Our results suggest that general cancer genes or proteins tend to be underexpressed in breast cancer tissue compared to healthy control tissue. Targeted mining for extracellular breast cancer proteins, on the other hand, can discover transcripts with over-expression in breast cancer tissues. Overexpression of a marker is key to developing a successful blood-based test for it because it is difficult to measure the absence of a marker. Based on our ovarian cancer results mentioned above, we believe that some transcripts code for proteins with the ability to discriminate women with cancer from those without, including cancers with poor outcome. We have developed protein assays for some of these and they are currently being validated in large sets of blood samples from women with breast cancer and healthy controls.

Markers of poor outcome

Half of the patients in our study had cancers with poor outcome. The patients had either died within 15 months of surgery, their cancer had recurred within 6 months or their cancer was of the basal-like subtype (triple negative for estrogen receptor, progesterone receptor and HER2). This allowed us to identify 21 markers for aggressive breast cancers in addition to those for all breast cancers. Of these, 17 genes were underexpressed in the poor-outcome cancers compared to the good-outcome cancers (Table 1). This is in accordance with breast cancer literature on differential gene expression between cancers with good and poor outcome,[57–61] where most of the transcripts were expressed lower in the cancers with less favorable outcome. Interestingly, these 17 transcripts show no differential expression between the cancer tissues with poor outcome and normal control tissues from healthy individuals, suggesting that, on the whole, molecular profiles might not be able to distinguish aggressive breast cancer tissue from healthy breast tissue. This suggests that the 17 genes have little potential as early detection markers for aggressive breast cancer, but they can be added to a rather large list of potential marker candidates for the prediction of breast cancer outcome. Although some of these genes have been linked to the basal subtype[61,62] and some are now being used to predict disease outcome, including *SCUBE2* in Oncotype DX[63] and Mammaprint,[57] the majority of them may constitute a novel group of genes that predict outcome and/or inform treatment.

Four genes were overexpressed in the cancers with poor outcome compared to both cancers with favorable outcome and healthy controls (Table 1). These are currently being investigated as potential blood

Table 1. Genes with differential expression in cancers with favorable as opposed to those with poor outcome[a]

Gene name	Expression
AR	L
CD44	L
CDKN1B	L
CFB	L
CTGF	L
EPOR	L
ERBB4	L
ESR1	L
ETAA1	L
FGFR2	L
FOXA1	L
GATA3	L
MMP10	H
MMP12	H
MMP2	L
MUC1	L
PGR	L
S100A7	H
SCUBE2	L
SPP1	H
TNFRSF10B	L

[a]L: Most genes are expressed at low levels in poor-outcome cancers compared to good-outcome cancers, but also at low levels in healthy controls. H: Four genes are expressed higher in poor-outcome cancers than in all other tissues. These are good potential markers for aggressive disease.

markers for early detection of cancers with poor outcome.

Markers expressed in cancer-surrounding normal tissue

Solid tumors cause many changes in the surrounding tissue. It is therefore likely that some potential biomarkers measure the body's response to cancer rather than processes in the cancer itself.[41] We further reason that molecular responses in the cancer-surrounding tissue can potentially be stronger than those in the cancers, particularly in the case of small lesions consisting of a few hundred cells. We base our assumption on findings by Tripathi and colleagues[54] and our own findings comparing breast cancer tissues to breast tissue from healthy individuals.[56] Tripathi and colleagues compared healthy tissue from breast reduction mammaplasties to normal tissue ipsilateral to the breast cancer and breast tissue with *in situ* disease. They found that global gene expression abnormalities exist in both normal epithelium of breast cancer patients and early cancers.[54]

Our own experiments[56] used cancer tissues that were scored for the proportion of viable tumor cells and supportive connective tissue (stroma) cells. The percentage of viable tumor cells varied from 30% to over 90%. Marker genes that are expressed in the cancer cells alone should therefore be able to separate the tissues with high tumor cell count from those with low count. Our findings, based on 71 transcripts, did not separate these two groups. Clustering patterns were rather based on disease outcome and on histology (Fig. 1).

Our findings resonate well with those of Tripathi and colleagues. We conclude that a cancer marker does not necessarily have to be expressed in the cancer cell alone. As stated initially, most breast cancer-related proteins were discovered from tumor cells, cell lines or mouse models. In their majority, these experiments did not use normal tissue or cells. Focusing on a comparison of normal, healthy state to the diseased state, possibly adding cancer-surrounding normal tissue, has the potential to benefit new marker discovery for the detection of breast cancer.

Markers for cancer predisposition of normal tissue

If the cancer influences its surrounding tissue, the same can be said about the opposite. Malignancy is a state that emerges from a tumor-host microenvironment[64] and it has been speculated that interactive signaling between tumor and stroma contributes to the formation of a complex multicellular organ.[65] Further, it has been debated whether molecular changes within the healthy tissue can promote transformation.[66] Thus, changes in the tumor environment could potentially precede cancer formation.

In our recent publication[56] we have discovered 33 breast cancer transcripts that are expressed in 20% of histologically normal tissue surrounding the breast cancer but not in healthy breast tissue (Table 2). We hypothesize that this signature could be an indicator for molecular predisposition of the normal breast tissue to cancer. We speculate that the sig-

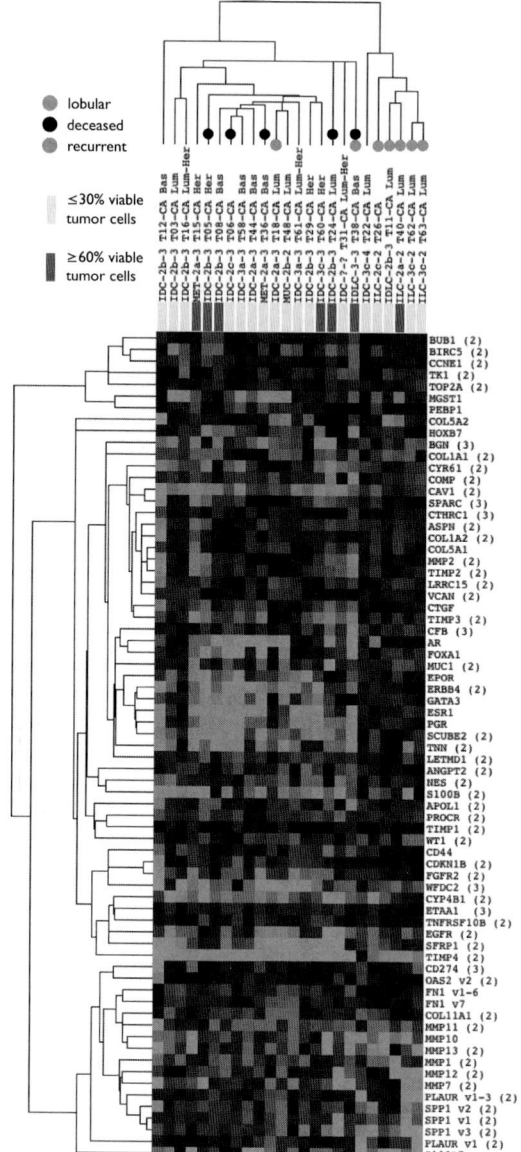

Figure 1. Viable tumor cell content does not influence clustering behavior. Unsupervised hierarchical clustering of 24 cancer tissues (17 with ≤30% viable tumor cells, yellow, and 7 with ≥60% viable tumor cells, red) and 71 transcripts. The lobular tumors are indicated with an orange dot. The tissues segregate based on histology (lobular vs. ductal) and disease outcome (patients who are deceased or have recurred vs. patients who have not). No clustering is observed based on tumor cell content of the tissue pieces used for real-time quantitative PCR.

nature, when expressed in otherwise healthy breast tissue could be an indicator of a precursor to a malignancy. As such it could be useful in patients with suspicious lesions where histological examination

Table 2. Thirty-three genes expressed in normal tissue from a breast with cancer whose expression pattern matches that of the cancer tissue[a]

Gene name	Expression
BGN	H
BIRC5	H
BUB1	H
CCNE1	H
CD274	H
COL11A1	H
COL1A1	H
COL1A2	H
COL5A1	H
COMP	H
CTHRC1	H
CYR61	L
EGFR	L
FN1	H
LETMD1	L
LRRC15	H
MMP1	H
MMP11	H
MMP13	H
NES	L
OAS2	H
PEBP1	L
PLAUR	H
PROCR	L
S100B	L
SFRP1	L
TIMP2	L
TK1	H
TNN	L
TOP2A	H
VCAN	H
WT1	H

[a]L: Genes with lower expression in cancer than in healthy breast control. H: Genes with higher expression in cancer than in healthy breast control.

of the biopsy is inconclusive. The signature could even be used independently of the histological information because we did not find any histological abnormality in the signature-expressing normal tissues ipsilateral to the breast cancer.

This signature could also be an indicator of disease severity if it is the result of the cancer influencing its environment. As such, the signature, when measured in normal tissue surrounding the breast cancer, could potentially predict disease outcome.

Finally, related to this, the occurrence of such cancer-predisposed normal tissue in women with a unilateral breast cancer could raise the odds of subsequent contralateral metachronous breast cancer in patients undergoing breast surgery. The ability to identify those individuals at greatest risk for a second primary breast cancer in the future would contribute to identification of patients who would benefit from total mastectomy (ipsilateral and/or contralateral) as opposed to breast-conserving surgery (lumpectomy).

Conclusions

Blood markers have the potential to complement mammography, thus improving its performance in screening. Blood markers can be discovered directly in blood but current methods are limited. Using the detour via the tissue transcriptome, a much larger number of markers can be discovered, but many of these will fail to retain their discriminatory power as proteins in blood. In spite of all recent effort in breast cancer marker research, relatively little is published on markers that discriminate healthy from cancerous breast tissues. We have shown that the inclusion of normal breast tissues from healthy individuals allowed us to identify novel tissue markers that are likely to work as protein blood markers, including some that are associated with aggressive disease or with predisposition to breast cancer.

Acknowledgments

Work was supported by DOD/CDMRP DAMD17-02-1-0691 and by NCI/Avon P50 CA083636.

Conflicts of interest

The authors declare no conflicts of interest.

References

1. American Cancer Society. 2010. Cancer Facts & Figures 2010. American Cancer Society. Atlanta, GA.
2. American Cancer Society. 2010. Breast Cancer Facts & Figures 2009–2010. American Cancer Society. Atlanta, GA.
3. Virnig, B.A, T.M. Tuttle, T. Shamliyan & R.L Kane. 2010. Ductal carcinoma in situ of the breast: a systematic review of incidence, treatment, and outcomes. *J. Natl. Cancer Inst.* **102:** 170–178.
4. Ernster, V.L. *et al.* 2002. Detection of ductal carcinoma in situ in women undergoing screening mammography. *J. Natl. Cancer Inst.* **94:** 1546–1554.

5. Kerlikowske, K., D. Grady, J. Barclay, *et al.* 1996. Likelihood ratios for modern screening mammography. Risk of breast cancer based on age and mammographic interpretation [see comments]. *JAMA* **276:** 39–43.

6. Carney, P.A *et al.* 2003. Individual and combined effects of age, breast density, and hormone replacement therapy use on the accuracy of screening mammography. *Ann. Intern. Med.* **138:** 168–175.

7. Bird, R.E., T.W. Wallace & B.C Yankaskas. 1992. Analysis of cancers missed at screening mammography. *Radiology.* **184:** 613–614.

8. Ma, L. *et al.* 1992. Case-control study of factors associated with failure to detect breast cancer by mammography [see comments]. *J. Natl. Cancer Inst.* **84:** 781–785.

9. Kerlikowske, K., D. Grady, J. Barclay, *et al.* 1996. Effect of age, breast density, and family history on the sensitivity of first screening mammography [see comments]. *JAMA* **276:** 33–38.

10. Esserman, L. *et al.* 2002. Improving the accuracy of mammography: volume and outcome relationships. *J. Natl. Cancer Inst.* **94:** 369–375.

11. Wegwarth, O. & G. Gigerenzer. 2010. "There is nothing to worry about": gynecologists' counseling on mammography. *Patient Educ. Couns.* **16:** 16.

12. Christiansen, C.L. *et al.* 2000. Predicting the cumulative risk of false-positive mammograms. *J. Natl. Cancer Inst.* **92:** 1657–1666.

13. Dean, P.B. & M. Pamilo. 1999. Screening mammography in Finland–1.5 million examinations with 97 percent specificity. Mammography Working Group, Radiological Society of Finland. *Acta Oncol.* **38**(Suppl 13): 47–54.

14. Elmore, J.G. *et al.* 1998. Ten-year risk of false positive screening mammograms and clinical breast examinations [see comments]. *N. Engl. J. Med.* **338:** 1089–1096.

15. Andersson, I. & L. Janzon. 1997. Reduced breast cancer mortality in women under age 50: updated results from the Malmö Mammographic Screening Program. *J. Natl. Cancer Inst. Monogr.* **22:** 63–67.

16. Gøtzsche, P.C & M. Nielsen. 2006. Screening for breast cancer with mammography. *Cochrane Database Syst. Rev.* **18:** Art. No. CD001877. doi:10.1002/14651858.CD001877.pub2.

17. Saslow, D. *et al.* 2007. American Cancer Society guidelines for breast screening with MRI as an adjunct to mammography. *CA Cancer J. Clin.* **57:** 75–89.

18. Day, D. 2009. Breast MRI: opportunities and challenges. *Minn. Med.* **92:** 45–48.

19. Lehman, C.D. *et al.* 2007. MRI evaluation of the contralateral breast in women with recently diagnosed breast cancer. *N. Engl. J. Med.* **356:** 1295–1303.

20. Swayampakula, A. K., Dillis, C. & Abraham, J. 2008. Role of MRI in screening, diagnosis and management of breast cancer. *Expert Rev. Anticancer Ther.* **8:** 811–817.

21. Heneghan, H.M. *et al.* 2010. Circulating microRNAs as novel minimally invasive biomarkers for breast cancer. *Ann. Surg.* **251:** 499–505.

22. Fassan, M. *et al.* 2009. MicroRNA expression profiling of male breast cancer. *Breast Cancer Res.* **11:** R58. doi:10.1186/bcr2348.

23. Cheung, K.L., A.J. Evans & J.F. Robertson. 2001. The use of blood tumour markers in the monitoring of metastatic breast cancer unassessable for response to systemic therapy. *Breast Cancer Res. Treat.* **67:** 273–278.

24. Cheung, K. L., Graves, C. R. & Robertson, J. F. 2000. Tumour marker measurements in the diagnosis and monitoring of breast cancer. *Cancer Treat. Rev.* **26:** 91–102.

25. Yonekubo, Y., Wu, P., Esechie, A., *et al.* 2010. Characterization of new serum biomarkers in breast cancer using lipid microarrays. *Tumour Biol.* **31:** 181–187.

26. Hammad, L.A. *et al.* 2009. Elevated levels of hydroxylated phosphocholine lipids in the blood serum of breast cancer patients. *Rapid Commun. Mass Spectrom.* **23:** 863–876.

27. Chajès, V. *et al.* 2008. Association between serum trans-monounsaturated fatty acids and breast cancer risk in the E3N-EPIC Study. *Am. J. Epidemiol.* **167:** 1312–1320.

28. Criscitiello, C., C. Sotiriou & M. Ignatiadis. 2010. Circulating tumor cells and emerging blood biomarkers in breast cancer. *Curr. Opin. Oncol.* 11 (Epub ahead of print). doi:10.1097/CCO.0b013e32833de186.

29. Ignatiadis, M., V. Georgoulias & D. Mavroudis. 2008. Circulating tumor cells in breast cancer. *Curr. Opin. Obstet. Gynecol.* **20:** 55–60.

30. Anderson, K.S. *et al.* 2010. p53 autoantibodies as potential detection and prognostic biomarkers in serous ovarian cancer. *Cancer Epidemiol. Biomarkers Prev.* **19:** 859–868.

31. Desmetz, C. *et al.* 2009. Identification of a new panel of serum autoantibodies associated with the presence of in situ carcinoma of the breast in younger women. *Clin. Cancer Res.* **15:** 4733–4741.

32. Yi, J.K. *et al.* 2009. Autoantibody to tumor antigen, alpha 2-HS glycoprotein: a novel biomarker of breast cancer screening and diagnosis. *Cancer Epidemiol. Biomarkers Prev.* **18:** 1357–1364.

33. Desmetz, C. *et al.* 2008. Proteomics-based identification of HSP60 as a tumor-associated antigen in early stage breast cancer and ductal carcinoma in situ. *J. Proteome Res.* **7:** 3830–3837.

34. Wang, F., Z. Zheng, J. Guo & X. Ding. 2010. Correlation and quantitation of microRNA aberrant expression in tissues and sera from patients with breast tumor. *Gynecol. Oncol.* 27 (Epub ahead of print). doi:10.1016/j.ygyno.2010.07.021.

35. Zoon, C.K. *et al.* 2009. Current molecular diagnostics of breast cancer and the potential incorporation of microRNA. *Expert Rev. Mol. Diagn.* **9:** 455–467.

36. Rui, Z., Jian-Guo, J., Yuan-Peng, T., *et al.* 2003. Use of serological proteomic methods to find biomarkers associated with breast cancer. *Proteomics* **3:** 433–439.

37. Wulfkuhle, J.D. *et al.* 2001. New approaches to proteomic analysis of breast cancer. *Proteomics.* **1:** 1205–1215.

38. Wulfkuhle, J.D. *et al.* 2002. Proteomics of human breast ductal carcinoma in situ. *Cancer Res.* **62:** 6740–6749.

39. Bouchal, P. *et al.* 2009. Biomarker discovery in low-grade breast cancer using isobaric stable isotope tags and two-dimensional liquid chromatography-tandem mass spectrometry (iTRAQ-2DLC-MS/MS) based quantitative proteomic analysis. *J. Proteome Res.* **8:** 362–373.

40. Belluco, C. *et al.* 2007. Serum proteomic analysis identifies a highly sensitive and specific discriminatory pattern in stage 1 breast cancer. *Ann. Surg. Oncol.* **14:** 2470–2476.

41. Jesneck, J.L *et al.* 2009. Do serum biomarkers really measure breast cancer? *BMC Cancer* **9:** 164. doi:10.1186/1471-2407-9-164.

42. Steiling, K. *et al.* 2009. Comparison of proteomic and transcriptomic profiles in the bronchial airway epithelium of current and never smokers. *PLoS ONE.* **4:** e5043. doi:10.1371/journal.pone.0005043.

43. Minagawa, H. *et al.* 2008. Comparative proteomic and transcriptomic profiling of the human hepatocellular carcinoma. *Biochem. Biophys. Res. Commun.* **366:** 186–192.

44. Hornshøj, H. *et al.* 2009. Transcriptomic and proteomic profiling of two porcine tissues using high-throughput technologies. *BMC Genomics.* **10:** 30. doi:10.1186/1471-2164-10-30.

45. Rogers, S. *et al.* 2008. Investigating the correspondence between transcriptomic and proteomic expression profiles using coupled cluster models. *Bioinformatics.* **24:** 2894–2900.

46. Glaesener, S. *et al.* 2008. Comparative proteome, transcriptome, and genome analysis of a gonadal and an extragonadal germ cell tumor cell line. *J. Proteome Res.* **7:** 3890–3899.

47. Van Der Auwera, I. *et al.* 2010. Integrated miRNA and mRNA expression profiling of the inflammatory breast cancer subtype. *Br. J. Cancer.* **103:** 532–541.

48. Schummer, M. *et al.* 1999. Comparative hybridization of an array of 21,500 ovarian cDNAs for the discovery of genes overexpressed in ovarian carcinomas. *Gene.* **238:** 375–385.

49. Palmer, C. *et al.* 2008. Systematic evaluation of candidate blood markers for detecting ovarian cancer. *PLoS ONE.* **3:** e2633. doi:10.1371/journal.pone.0002633.

50. Lowe, K.A. *et al.* 2008. Effects of Personal Characteristics on Serum CA125, Mesothelin, and HE4 Levels in Healthy Postmenopausal Women at High-Risk for Ovarian Cancer. *Cancer Epidemiol. Biomarkers Prev.* **17:** 2480–2487. doi: 17/9/2480 [pii], 10.1158/1055-9965.EPI-08-0150.

51. McIntosh, M. *et al.* 2004. Combining CA 125 and SMR serum markers for diagnosis and early detection of ovarian carcinoma. *Gynecol. Oncol.* **95:** 9–15.

52. Shah, C.A *et al.* 2009. Influence of ovarian cancer risk status on the diagnostic performance of the serum biomarkers Mesothelin, HE4, and CA125. *Cancer Epidemiol. Biomarkers Prev.* **18:** 1365–1372.

53. Köhrmann, A., Kammerer, U., Kapp, M., *et al.* 2009. Expression of matrix metalloproteinases (MMPs) in primary human breast cancer and breast cancer cell lines: new findings and review of the literature. *BMC Cancer* **9:** 188, doi: 1471-2407-9-188 [pii], 10.1186/1471–2407-9-188.

54. Tripathi, A. *et al.* 2008. Gene expression abnormalities in histologically normal breast epithelium of breast cancer patients. *Int. J. Cancer.* **122:** 1557–1566. doi: 10.1002/ijc.23267.

55. Bièche, I. *et al.* 2004. Molecular profiling of inflammatory breast cancer: identification of a poor-prognosis gene expression signature. *Clin. Cancer Res.* **10:** 6789–6795. doi: 10/20/6789 [pii], 10.1158/1078-0432.CCR-04-0306.

56. Schummer, M. *et al.* 2010. Comparison of breast cancer to healthy control tissue discovers novel markers with potential for prognosis and early detection. *PLoS ONE.* **5:** e9122. doi:10.1371/journal.pone.0009122.

57. van 't Veer, L.J. *et al.* 2002. Gene expression profiling predicts clinical outcome of breast cancer. *Nature.* **415:** 530–536.

58. van 't Veer, L. *et al.* 2003. Expression profiling predicts outcome in breast cancer. *Breast Cancer Res.* **5:** 57–58. doi: 10.1186/bcr562.

59. van de Vijver, M.J *et al.* 2002. A gene-expression signature as a predictor of survival in breast cancer. *N. Engl. J. Med.* **347:** 1999–2009.

60. Sørlie, T. *et al.* 2001. Gene expression patterns of breast carcinomas distinguish tumor subclasses with clinical implications. *Proc. Natl. Acad. Sci. USA* **98:** 10869–10874.

61. Sørlie, T. *et al.* 2003. Repeated observation of breast tumor subtypes in independent gene expression data sets. *Proc. Natl. Acad. Sci. USA* **100:** 8418–8423.

62. Perou, C.M *et al.* 2000. Molecular portraits of human breast tumours. *Nature.* **406:** 747–752.

63. Paik, S. *et al.* 2004. A multigene assay to predict recurrence of tamoxifen-treated, node-negative breast cancer. *N. Engl. J. Med.* **351:** 2817–2826.

64. Wernert, N. 1997. The multiple roles of tumour stroma. *Virchows Arch.* **430:** 433–443.

65. Mueller, M.M. & N.E Fusenig. 2004. Friends or foes—bipolar effects of the tumour stroma in cancer. *Nat. Rev. Cancer.* **4:** 839–849.

66. Liotta, L.A. & E.C Kohn. 2001. The microenvironment of the tumour-host interface. *Nature.* **411:** 375–379.

Ann. N.Y. Acad. Sci. ISSN 0077-8923

ANNALS OF THE NEW YORK ACADEMY OF SCIENCES
Issue: *Toward Personalized Medicine for Cancer*

Novel anti-fatty acid synthase compounds with anti-cancer activity in HER2+ breast cancer

G. Oliveras,[1] A. Blancafort,[1] A. Urruticoechea,[2] O. Campuzano,[1] D. Gómez-Cabello,[3] R. Brugada,[1] M. L. López-Rodríguez,[4] R. Colomer,[3] and T. Puig[1]

[1]Institut d'Investigació Biomèdica de Girona – Facultat de Medicina, Girona, Spain. [2]Institut Català d'Oncologia, Institut d'Investigació Biomèdica de Bellvitge, Barcelona, Spain. [3]Centro Oncológico MD Anderson España, Madrid, Spain. [4]Química Orgánica I, Facultad de Ciencias Químicas, Universidad Complutense, Madrid, Spain

Address for correspondence: Teresa Puig, Institut d'Investigació Biomèdica de Girona, Universitat de Girona, Girona, Spain. mtpuig@iconcologia.net

Fatty acid synthase (FASN) expression and activity has emerged as a common phenotype in most human carcinomas, including breast cancer, and its expression is tightly linked to HER2 signaling pathways. The development of inhibitors of FASN activity has consequently appeared as a novel antitarget modality for treating cancer. However, the clinical use of FASN inhibitors, such as cerulenin, C75, and epigallocatechin 3-gallate (EGCG), is limited by anorexia and induced body weight loss or by its low *in vivo* potency and stability. Here, we summarize the design and development of G28UCM, the lead-compound of a novel family of synthetic FASN inhibitors, with both *in vitro* and *in vivo* activity in a human breast cancer model of FASN+ and HER2+.

Keywords: breast cancer; fatty acid synthase (FASN); novel anti-FASN compounds; HER2; preclinical study

New approaches to cancer treatment: lipogenesis and cancer

Since the 1920s, cancer cells have been known to exhibit an altered metabolism; currently, it is known that this point is crucial for both cancer cell survival and anticancer drug development. One hallmark of malignant cells is their higher rate of energy-consuming processes due to the increased protein and DNA synthesis needed to maintain cell division.[1] In 1924, Warburg and colleagues observed that cancer cells consume glucose through an anaerobic pathway in order to produce lactic acid (the Warburg effect),[2] providing malignant cells with an advantage in the tumor microenvironment.[3] This enhanced anaerobic glycolysis produces an excess of pyruvate that is transformed into lactate and acetyl-CoA. The high proliferation ratio of cancer cells increases their need for fatty acids (FA) as substrates for the biosynthesis of phospholipids, which are essential constituents of biological membranes and are involved in protein acylation and energy production through β-oxidation.[4]

FA are present as metabolic substrates in normal cells and are restored as triglycerides (TG) in adipose tissue. The body's pool of FA comes from different sources, both exogenous (e.g., dietary FA) and endogenous, including both the hydrolysis of TG (from adipose tissue) and the lipogenic pathway (*de novo* synthesis). Thus, this constitutes one of the important metabolic differences between normal and cancer cells. While most human tissues prefer using exogenous lipids for the synthesis of new structural lipids (including phospholipids, TG, and cholesterol esters), and so fatty acid synthase (FASN) expression is low, it has been reported that in cancer cells, FA were derived mainly from *de novo* synthesis.[5] The imperative need of cancer cells to synthesize FA has promoted the selection of two regulatory enzymes—FASN and acetyl-CoA carboxylase (ACC)—and one intermediate enzyme, malonyl-CoA, as drugable targets as a new approach to cancer treatment. Accordingly, FASN expression and activity have emerged as a common phenotype in most human cancer cells and is mostly absent in the corresponding normal cells.[6] Since the 1990s,

doi: 10.1111/j.1749-6632.2010.05777.x

mounting evidence has pointed to an important role of FASN in cancer cell survival, progression, and malignancy. FASN has emerged as a prognosis biomarker in breast, prostate, and other carcinomas and we have shown that its inhibition is specifically cytotoxic for human cancer cells.[5,7] Although part of these effects could be due to the accumulation of malonyl-CoA,[8] similar effects have been observed by inhibiting other lipogenic enzymes, suggesting that lipogenesis has an important role in the cancer physiopathology.[9] In summary, FASN plays an essential role in energy homeostasis and could be a good target for the development of both anti-obesity and anticancer agents.

FASN expression and regulation in normal and cancer cells

FASN (E.C.2.3.1.85) is a homodimeric multienzymatic protein of 250–270kD divided into seven functional domains, assembled into two homodimers.[10] Through a series of 32 reactions, FASN is able to synthesize long chain fatty acids (LCFA), mainly palmitate, using acetyl-CoA and malonyl-CoA as substrates and NADPH as an electron donor.[11]

FASN is expressed mainly in lipogenic tissues, in some hormone-sensitive cells (e.g., lactating mammary glands, cycling endometrium, and seminal vesicles), in various specialized cell types (type II alveolar cells to produce surfactant, hypothalamus to control food intake), and in proliferating fetal cells.[12,13] In adults, lipogenesis is required primarily for the following: (1) to store excess of energy ingested as carbohydrates by generating TG; (2) to synthesize fat from other substrates (carbohydrate or protein) in fat-deficient diets; or (3) to produce FA in special tissues or situations such as the synthesis of medium chain fatty acids in lactation. Taking into account these functions, the role of FASN in a well-nourished population is not of great significance, as dietary lipids cover the requirements to maintain homeostasis.[14] In normal cells, FASN expression remains at low levels and its regulation is complex and highly dependent on nutritional status and on the hormonal profile.[11] To summarize, FASN is activated by nutritional status and its expression is mediated by different signaling pathways, such as the phosphoinositide-3 kinase/protein kinase B (PI3K/Akt) and mitogen-activated protein kinase/extracellular signal-regulated kinase (MAPK/

ERK1/2) pathways that modulate the expression and maturation status of the transcriptional factor sterol response element binding proteins (SREBP-1) to produce SREBP-1c, which modulates FASN gene maturation and expression[15] (Fig. 1A).

The first signal that FA in cancer cells were due to *de novo* synthesis was sent out in the 1950s, when Medes and colleagues[16] determined that most of the FA esterified in tumors were FASN products (approximately 93% of FA originated from TG). In general, cancer cells are characterized by an exacerbated anaerobic glycolysis accompanied by an activation of the glycolytic enzymes[2] and also by an increased level of synthesis of FA that correlates with an overexpression and hyperactivity of lipogenic enzymes such as FASN.[17] This phenotype seems to give to malignant cells an advantage for survival and growth in the microenvironment of biological and metabolic tumors.[18] FASN overexpression and hyperactivation have been described in many cancers and commonly correlate with a higher rate of recurrence and a lower chance of survival.[19] Using immunohistochemistry analysis, high levels of FASN have been observed in many preneoplasic lesions, including breast, pancreas, prostate, colon, and lung cancer. The pathways responsible for FASN overexpression in cancer cells are not yet well understood. Four different mechanisms have been proposed: enhanced transcription, increased translation, greater stability of proteins, and gene amplification.[7] These mechanisms may be active at the same time and may prevent FASN from its physiological regulation, thus resulting in a constitutive activation of the lipogenic pathway in tumors. FASN regulation at the transcriptional level is one of the most studied mechanisms. It involves mainly growth factors/growth factor receptors (GF/GFR) and steroid hormones/steroid hormone receptors (SH/SHR), although new players such as hypoxia-inducible factor 1 (HIF-1α) and p53 family members have recently been implied in the regulation of FASN expression. It is important to notice that at the transcriptional level, the expression of FASN in both normal and cancer cells occurs in most cases through the same signaling pathways (PI3K/AKT/mTOR and MAPK/ERK1/2) by promoting the binding of SREBP-1c to its responding elements in the FASN promoter. The main difference between normal and cancer cells is the stimuli that activate the signaling cascades (Fig. 1B).

A

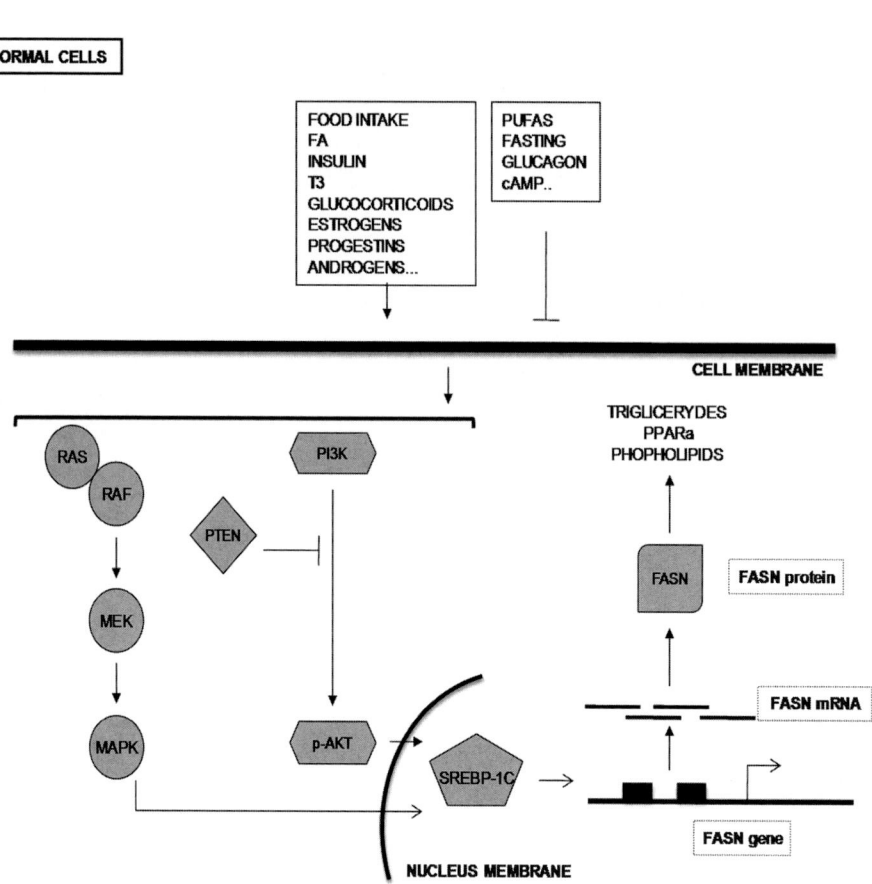

Figure 1. FASN regulation in normal and cancer cells. (A) FASN expression in normal cells is dependent on nutritional and hormonal status. FASN transcription is upregulated by food intake, fatty acids (FA), or hormones and downregulated by polyunsaturated fatty acids (PUFAS), cAMP, or fasting (glucagon). These stimuli activate different cascades, such as the phosphoinositide 3-kinase/protein kinase B (PI3K/AKT) or mitogen-activated protein kinase/extracellular signal regulated kinase (MAPK/ERK1/2) pathways, which finally modulate the expression and maturation status of the sterol regulatory element-binding protein 1C (SREBP-1C). The active form of SREBP1C is translocated into the nucleus where it can bind to the FASN promoter responding elements. (B) In cancer cells, the growth factors (GF) or steroid hormones (SH)—esterols, androgens or progesterone—lead, through their receptors (GFR/SHR), to downstream PI3K/AKT, MAPK/ERK1/2, or mTOR signaling pathways by, finally, promoting the binding of SREBP-1C to its responding elements in the FASN promoter region. FASN expression in cancer cells is also activated by the tumor microenvironment (hypoxia and acidosis) through the upregulation of the hypoxia-inducible factor 1α (HIF-1α), which induces the AKT activation. Other proteins, such as p53 or SPOT14, are able to increase FASN transcription. FASN expression can also be achieved at the posttranslational level through interaction with USP2a, a preproteasomal ubiquitin-specific protease that, by removing ubiquitin from FASN, strongly stabilizes FASN protein. All these pathways can occur simultaneously in cancer cells. (Figure taken from Relat & Puig.[41])

In cancer cells, FASN is insensitive to nutritional signals and SREBP-1c expression and activation is driven by aberrant GF/GFR and SH/SHR levels or impaired signaling pathways.[5,18]

FASN: a biomarker and a druggable target

FASN expression and activity have been shown to be a common phenotype in most human tumor cells, and it has been demonstrated that FASN plays an essential role in tumor growth and survival.[20] In prostate and breast cancer, several studies have demonstrated an association between FASN expression and the prognosis of the disease. In stage I breast cancer, patients with high levels of FASN show a fourfold increased risk of death from this pathology than patients with lower FASN protein levels.[21] In

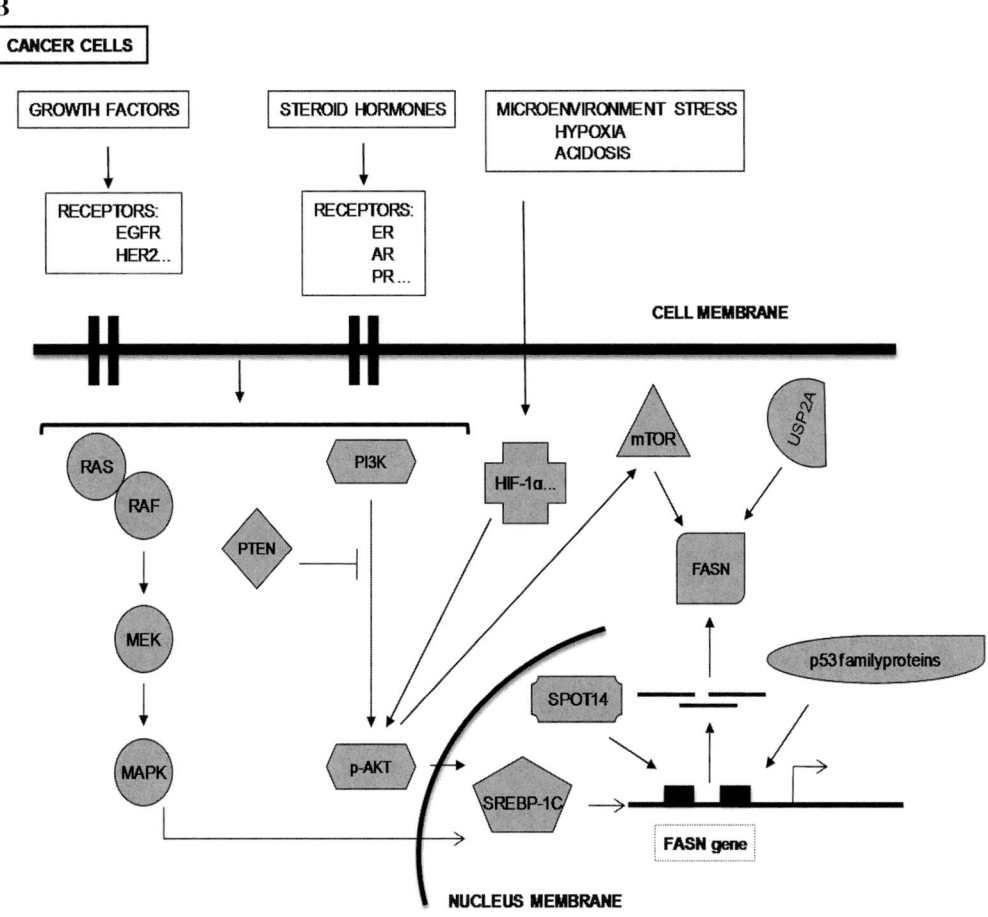

Figure 1. *Continued.*

prostate cancer, FASN expression correlates with a fourfold risk of recurrence and an increased Gleason grade and risk of death from the disease. It has been shown that this risk raises up to 12-fold when PTEN is deleted.[22] FASN expression has also been associated with HER2 expression in poor prognosis tumors.[23] Recently, an ELISA assay has been developed to show the positive correlation between circulating levels of FASN and the disease's degree.[24] However, further studies will be necessary to deepen in the role of FASN expression in the cancer prognosis and the usefulness of determining FASN in serum or in tumor samples as pathologic markers for diagnoses or for predicting the progression of the disease.

Recent studies have sought to describe the effect of FASN activity inhibition on the cell cycle status. The fact is that the disruption of *de novo* FA synthesis

impairs their DNA synthesis and cell cycle progression. Many efforts have been made into developing pharmacological anti-FASN activity compounds. At a molecular level, different pathways have been modified by FASN inhibition and it has been shown that cancer cell death can also be increased if FASN inhibitors are combined with inhibitors of FASN-related signaling cascades (e.g., PI3K/AKT, HER2, and mTOR).[22,25] In addition to cell arrest, FASN inhibition causes cancer cell death.[26] The inhibition of FA synthesis using siRNA against FASN or ACC reduces the incorporation of phospholipids into membranes, causing morphological changes in cells and ultimately leading to apoptosis of breast and prostate cancer cells without affecting nonmalignant cells.[8] It has been observed that FASN inhibition (using siRNAs or small molecules) causes ER stress and activation of an unfolded protein

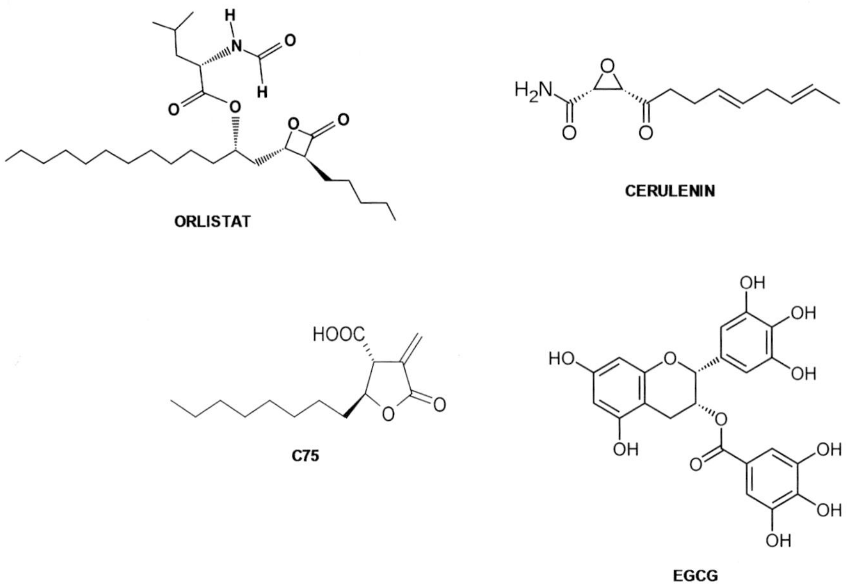

Figure 2. Chemical structure of the FASN inhibitors.

response (UPR), inducing cell death.[27] FASN inhibition also causes an increase of malonyl-CoA levels that could result in an accumulation of malonyl-CoA or toxic lipid intermediates that finally induce cell death.[8] Finally, FASN overexpression is associated with the palmitoylation of signaling proteins, so that the interference of this pathway may also induce apoptosis.[28]

In summary, many reasons point to FASN as a novel druggable target against cancer. Thus, many efforts have been put toward developing inhibitors of FASN activity as novel anticancer compounds, alone or combined with other anticancer drugs.

Preclinical development of FASN inhibitors

The most studied FASN inhibitors are cerulenin and its synthetic derivative C75 (Fig. 2). Cerulenin [2S,3R)-2,3-epoxi-4-oxo-7,10-dodecadien oxylamide] is a mycotoxin metabolite derived from *Cephalosporium caerulens*,[14] which covalently blocks the β-ketoacyl synthase activity (KS) of FASN, thus avoiding condensation between the acyl intermediate and malonyl-CoA. It has been reported that cerulenin is able to delay the progression of breast, ovarian, and prostate human cancer xenografts.[29] Because of the cerulenin chemical instability caused by a reactive epoxi group and the poor systemic availability of cerulenin, two

structurally related synthetic molecules were developed: C75 and C93.[26,29] C75 is a cerulenin-derived compound that lacks the reactive epoxi group (Fig. 2).[29] C75 was initially synthesized as an inhibitor of mammalian FASN and structurally related to malonyl-CoA. Although initially it provides the first evidence of *in vivo* growth tumor reduction after FASN inhibition,[29] its clinical development as an antitumor agent has been discarded owing to the side effects produced. The use of C75 *in vivo* is limited by anorexia and body weight loss, which we and others have associated with the stimulation of carnitine palmitoyltransferase-1 (CPT-1), the enzyme responsible for the regulation of mitochondrial fatty acid oxidation.[30] C93 is a C75 analogue that blocks the KS domain of FASN without stimulating FA oxidation or causing body weight loss.[31] This improvement makes it possible to treat animals more frequently than with C75 and also increases the effectiveness of the treatment. Another advantage of C93 is that it can be administered orally.[32] Orlistat is a β-lactone that was first approved as an anti-obesity drug. Orlistat targets gastrointestinal lipases and inhibits FASN by blocking its TE activity domain, which is responsible for releasing palmitate.[33] Although it has been demonstrated that Orlistat inhibits the growth of a prostate tumor xenograft,[34] its poor solubility and bioavailability seem to limit the

Table 1. Structure and biological activity of novel polyphenolic compound

Compound	EGCG		G28UCM	Inhibition of FASN activity (% of control)
	Cancer cell cytotoxicity (IC$_{50}$ (μM)) [FASN/HER2 expression levels]			
	AU565 [+++]	MCF-7 [+]	MDA-MB-231 [$\pm$]	
EGCG	190 ± 20	205 ± 7	197 ± 15	20
G28UCM	30 ± 5	46 ± 18	79 ± 4	90

use of orlistat as an antitumor drug. It has also been observed that Orlistat suppresses endothelial cell proliferation and angiogenesis by inhibiting FASN.[35]

Polyphenols constitute a wide group of different molecular structures: catechins, flavones, anthocyanidins, anthraquinones, lignans, coumarins, and tannins. Some tea polyphenols (black tea and green tea) are able to control body weight, inhibit cancer cell growth, diminish fat accumulation in the liver and blood, and act as antioxidants. These polyphenols function through many different mechanisms, including the following: inducing apoptosis, stimulating lipid metabolism, inhibiting lipases, regulating thermogenesis, controlling food intake, and blocking FASN activity.[35]

Polyphenolic catechins are the main components of green tea and include epicatechin (EC), epicatechin 3-gallate (ECG), epigallo-catechin (EGC), and epigallocatechin-3-gallate (EGCG), which is considered the main player in relation to the therapeutic properties of green tea and is also the most abundant variety (Fig. 2). Recent studies have reported that EGCG, the main polyphenolic catechin of green tea, and other naturally occurring flavonoids (such as luteolin, quercetin, and kaempferol) inhibit FASN, induce apoptosis of several tumor cell lines *in vitro*, and reduce the size of mammary tumors in animal models.[36] We have recently reported a simultaneous comparison of the cellular, molecular, and functional effects on the key fatty acid metabolism enzymes FASN and CPT-1 of C75 versus EGCG in breast cancer cells.[9,37,38] We showed that EGCG achieves all cellular, functional, and molecular antitumor effects of known FASN inhibitors but, unlike C75, it did not increase CPT-1 activity. However, the *in vivo* effect of EGCG might be limited by its IC$_{50}$ value, as well as its relative instability under the slightly neutral or alkaline physiological

conditions,[13] which may be illustrated by the limited activity of green tea in prostate cancer clinical trials. Based on the chemical structure of EGCG, we have recently reported the synthesis and biological evaluation of a new series of polyphenolic derivatives, which has resulted in the identification of two potent FASN inhibitors with high antitumor activity *in vitro*.[39] Novel compounds were selected based on their FASN activity inhibition and their selective cancer cell cytoxicity in a panel of human breast cancer cells composed by AU565, MCF-7, and MDA-MB-231, as *in vitro* models of high (+++), moderate (+), and low ($\pm$) levels of FASN expression, respectively. We observed that two of the novel polyphenolic compounds were quite superior to EGCG in terms of cancer cytotoxicity and FASN activity inhibition.[40] Among them, G28UCM was selected because of its high FASN activity inhibition, its potent and selective cancer cell cytotoxicity (Table 1), its ability to induce apoptosis in a FASN/HER2+ breast cancer model, and finally its marked inhibition of HER2-related signaling pathways compared to EGCG.[40] We have preformed preliminary experiments to evaluate the pharmacological interaction between G28UCM and different anti-HER agents against FASN$^+$ and HER2$^+$ breast cancer cells (AU565 cells), and the potential effectiveness of G28UCM in an *in vivo* animal study of breast cancer FASN$^+$/HER2$^+$ xenograft. Preliminary results indicate that intraperitoneal G28UCM treatment (40 mg/kg/day) of animals exhibited marked tumor volume reduction compared with the vehicle treated control animals without any changes in FASN protein expression analyzed by immunohistochemistry. Importantly, no significant weight loss or anorexia was identified after 45 days of daily G28UCM-treatment in the experimental group. Hematoxylin-eosin and picrosirius red stains of the myocardium showed no significant structural alterations between the control and G28UCM-treated animals (work in progress). Our preliminary findings provide a rationale for the preclinical development of G28UCM, alone or in combination, as a suitable new agent for treating HER2-overexpressing breast cancer.

Conflicts of interest

The authors declare no conflicts of interest.

References

1. Clemens, M.J. 2004. Targets and mechanisms for the regulation of translation in malignant transformation. *Oncogene* **23:** 3180–3188.
2. Warburg, O. 1956. On the origin of cancer cells. *Science* **123:** 309–314.
3. Kuhajda, F.P. 2000. Fatty-acid Synthase and human cancer: new perspectives on its role in tumor biology. *Nutrition* **16:** 202–208.
4. Kuhajda, F.P. 2006. Fatty acid synthase and cancer: new application of an old pathway. *Cancer Res.* **66:** 5977–5980.
5. Milgraum, F.P., L.A. Witters, G.R. Pasternack & F.P. Kuhajda. 1997. Enzymes of the fatty acid synthesis pathway are highly expressed in situ breast carcinoma. *Clin. Cancer Res.* **3:** 2115–2120.
6. Swinnen, J.V., K. Brusselmans & G. Verhoeven. 2006. Increased lipogenesis in cancer cells: new players, novel targets. *Curr. Opin. Clin. Nutr. Metab. Care.* **9:** 358–365.
7. Thupari, J.N., M.L. Pinn & F.P. Kuhajda. 2001. Fatty acid synthase inhibition in human breast cancer cells leads to malonyl-CoA-induced inhibition of fatty acid oxidation and cytotoxicity. *Biochem. Biophys. Res. Commun.* **285:** 217–223.
8. Brusselmans, K., E. De Schrijver, G. Verhoeven & J.V. Swinnen. 2005. RNA interference mediated silencing of the acetyl-CoA-carboxylase-alpha gene induces growth inhibition and apoptosis of prostate cancer cells. *Cancer Res.* **65:** 6719–6725.
9. Smith, S. 1994. The animal fatty acid synthase: one gene, one polypeptide, seven enzymes. *FASEB J.* **8:** 1248–1259.
10. Little, J.L. & S.J. Kridel. 2008. Fatty acid synthase activity in tumor cells. *Subcell. Biochem.* **49:** 169–194.
11. Kusakabe, T., M. Maeda, N. Hoshi, *et al.* 2000. Fatty acid synthase is expressed mainly in adult hormone-sensitive cells or cells with high lipid metabolism and in proliferating fetal cells. *Histochem. Cytochem.* **48:** 613–622.
12. López, M., C.J. Lelliott & A. Vidal-Puig. 2007. Hypothalamic fatty acid metabolism: a housekeeping pathway that regulates food intake. *Bioessays* **29:** 248–261.
13. Weiss, L., G.E. Hoffmann, R. Schreiber, *et al.* 1986. Fatty-acid biosynthesis in man, a pathway of minor importance: purification, optimal assay conditions, and organ distribution of fatty-acid synthase. *Biol. Chem. Hoppe Seyler* **367:** 905–912.
14. Porstmann, T., B. Griffiths, Y.L. Chung, *et al.* 2005. PKB/Akt induces transcription of enzymes involved in cholesterol and fatty acid biosynthesis via activation of SREBP. *Oncogene* **24:** 6465–6481.
15. Medes, G., A. Thomas & S. Weinhouse. 1953. Metabolism of neoplastic tissue IV: a study of lipid synthesis in neoplastic tissue slices in vitro. *Cancer Res.* **13:** 27–29.
16. Szutowicz, A., J. Kwiatkowski & S. Angielski. 1979. Lipogenetic and glycolytic enzyme activities in carcinoma and non-malignant diseases of the human breast. *Br. J. Cancer* **39:** 681–687.
17. Menendez, J.A. & R. Lupu. 2007. Fatty acid synthase and the lipogenic phenotype in cancer pathogenesis. *Nat. Rev. Cancer* **7:** 763–777.
18. Visca, P., V. Sebastiani, C. Botti, *et al.* 2004. Fatty acid synthase (FASN) is a marker of increased risk of recurrence in lung carcinoma. *Anticancer Res.* **24:** 4169–4173.
19. Puig, T., R. Porta & R. Colomer. 2009. Fatty acid synthase: a new anti-tumor target. *Med. Clin.* **132:** 359–363.
20. Wang, Y., F.P. Kuhajda, J.N. Li, *et al.* 2001. Fatty acid synthase (FASN) expression in human breast cancer cell culture supernatants and in breast cancer patients. *Cancer Lett.* **167:** 99–104.
21. Bandyopadhyay, S., S.K. Pai, M. Watabe, *et al.* 2005. FASN expression inversely correlates with PTEN level in prostate cancer and a PI 3-kinase inhibitor synergizes with FASN siRNA to induce apoptosis. *Oncogene* **24:** 5389–5395.
22. Zhang, D., L.K. Tai, L.L. Wong, *et al.* 2005. Proteomic study reveals that proteins involved in metabolic and detoxification pathways are highly expressed in HER2/neupositive breast cancer. *Mol. Cell Proteomics* **4:** 1686–1696.
23. Wang, Y., F.P. Kuhajda, L.J. Sokoll & D.W. Chan. 2001. Two-site ELISA for the quantitative determination of fatty acid synthase. *Clin. Chim. Acta.* **304:** 107–115.
24. Liu, X., Y. Shi, V.L. Giranda & Y. Luo. 2006. Inhibition of the phosphatidylinositol 3-kinase/Akt pathway sensitizes MDA MB468 human breast cancer cells to cerulenin-induced apoptosis. *Mol. Cancer Ther.* **5:** 494–501.
25. Pizer, E.S., C. Jackisch, F.D. Wood, *et al.* 1996. Inhibition of fatty acid synthesis induces programmed cell death in human breast cancer cells. *Cancer Res.* **56:** 2745–2747.
26. Little, J.L., F.B. Wheeler, D.R. Fels, *et al.* 2007. Inhibition of fatty acid synthase induces endoplasmic reticulum stress in tumor cells. *Cancer Res.* **67:** 1262–1269.
27. Fiorentino, M., G. Zadra, E. Palescandolo, *et al.* 2008. Overexpression of fatty acid synthase is associated with palmitoylation of Wnt1 and cytoplasmic stabilization of beta-catenin in prostate cancer. *Lab. Invest.* **88:** 1340–1348.
28. Kuhajda, F.P., E.S. Pizer, J.N. Li, *et al.* 2000. Synthesis and antitumor activity of an inhibitor of fatty acid synthase. *Proc. Natl. Acad. Sci. USA* **97:** 3450–3454.
29. Wortman, M.D., D.J. Clegg, D. D'Alessio, *et al.* 2003. C75 inhibits food intake by increasing CNS glucose metabolism. *Nat. Med.* **9:** 483–485.
30. Orita, H., J. Coulter, C. Lemmon, *et al.* 2007. Selective inhibition of fatty acid synthase for lung cancer treatment. *Clin. Cancer Res.* **13:** 7139–7145.
31. Orita, H., J. Coulter, E. Tully, *et al.* 2008. Inhibiting fatty acid synthase for chemoprevention of chemically induced lung tumors. *Clin. Cancer Res.* **14:** 2458–2464.
32. Kridel, S.J., F. Axelrod, N. Rozenkrantz & J.W. Smith. 2004. Orlistat is a novel inhibitor of fatty acid synthase with anti-tumor activity. *Cancer Res.* **64:** 2070–2075.
33. Menendez, J.A., L. Vellon & R. Lupu. 2005. Orlistat: from antiobesity drug to anticancer agent in Her-2/neu

(erbB-2)-overexpressing gastrointestinal tumors? *Exp. Biol. Med.* **230:** 151–154.

34. Browne, C.D., E.J. Hindmarsh & J.W. Smith. 2006. Inhibition of endothelial cell proliferation and angiogenesis by orlistat, a fatty acid synthase inhibitor. *FASEB J.* **20:** 2027–2035.

35. Lin, J.K. & S.Y. Lin-Shiau. 2006. Mechanisms of hypolipidemic and anti-obesity effects of tea and tea polyphenols. *Mol. Nutr. Food Res.* **50:** 211–217.

36. Jatoi, A., N. Ellison, P.A. Burch, *et al.* 2003. A phase II trial of green tea in the treatment of patients with androgen independent metastatic prostate carcinoma. *Cancer* **97:** 1442–1446.

37. Puig, T., A. Vázquez-Martín, J. Relat, *et al.* 2008. Fatty acid metabolism in breast cancer cells: differential inhibitory ef-

fects of epigallocatechin gallate (EGCG) and C75. *Breast Cancer Res. Treat.* **109:** 471–479.

38. Puig, T., J. Relat, P.F. Marrero, *et al.* 2008. Green tea catechin inhibits fatty acid synthase without stimulating carnitine palmitoyltransferase-1 or inducing weight loss in experimental animals. *Anticancer Res.* **28:** 3671–3676.

39. Colomer, R., T. Puig, J. Brunet, *et al.* 2007. Novel polyhydroxylated compounds as fatty acid synthase (FASN) inhibitors. European Patent EP07110956.5.

40. Puig, T., C. Turrado, B. Benhamú, *et al.* 2009. Novel Inhibitors of Fatty Acid Synthase with Anticancer Activity. *Clin Cancer Res.* **15:** 7608–7615.

41. Relat, J. & T. Puig. 2010. *Frontiers in Drug Design and Discovery.* **5:** 211–235.